CN-54 CERTIFIED NURSE EXAMINATION SERIES

This is your
PASSBOOK for...

Certified Long Term Care Nurse

Test Preparation Study Guide
Questions & Answers

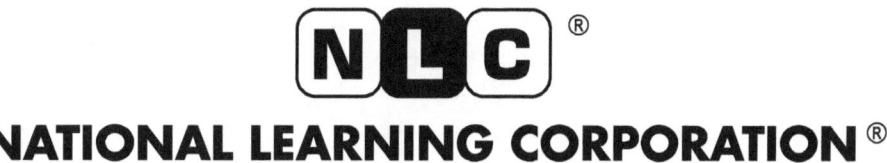

COPYRIGHT NOTICE

This book is SOLELY intended for, is sold ONLY to, and its use is RESTRICTED to individual, bona fide applicants or candidates who qualify by virtue of having seriously filed applications for appropriate license, certificate, professional and/or promotional advancement, higher school matriculation, scholarship, or other legitimate requirements of education and/or governmental authorities.

This book is NOT intended for use, class instruction, tutoring, training, duplication, copying, reprinting, excerption, or adaptation, etc., by:

1) Other publishers
2) Proprietors and/or Instructors of "Coaching" and/or Preparatory Courses
3) Personnel and/or Training Divisions of commercial, industrial, and governmental organizations
4) Schools, colleges, or universities and/or their departments and staffs, including teachers and other personnel
5) Testing Agencies or Bureaus
6) Study groups which seek by the purchase of a single volume to copy and/or duplicate and/or adapt this material for use by the group as a whole without having purchased individual volumes for each of the members of the group
7) Et al.

Such persons would be in violation of appropriate Federal and State statutes.

PROVISION OF LICENSING AGREEMENTS – Recognized educational, commercial, industrial, and governmental institutions and organizations, and others legitimately engaged in educational pursuits, including training, testing, and measurement activities, may address request for a licensing agreement to the copyright owners, who will determine whether, and under what conditions, including fees and charges, the materials in this book may be used them. In other words, a licensing facility exists for the legitimate use of the material in this book on other than an individual basis. However, it is asseverated and affirmed here that the material in this book CANNOT be used without the receipt of the express permission of such a licensing agreement from the Publishers. Inquiries re licensing should be addressed to the company, attention rights and permissions department.

All rights reserved, including the right of reproduction in whole or in part, in any form or by any means, electronic or mechanical, including photocopying, recording, or by any information storage and retrieval system, without permission in writing from the Publisher.

Copyright © 2024 by
National Learning Corporation

212 Michael Drive, Syosset, NY 11791
(516) 921-8888 • www.passbooks.com
E-mail: info@passbooks.com

PASSBOOK® SERIES

THE *PASSBOOK® SERIES* has been created to prepare applicants and candidates for the ultimate academic battlefield – the examination room.

At some time in our lives, each and every one of us may be required to take an examination – for validation, matriculation, admission, qualification, registration, certification, or licensure.

Based on the assumption that every applicant or candidate has met the basic formal educational standards, has taken the required number of courses, and read the necessary texts, the *PASSBOOK® SERIES* furnishes the one special preparation which may assure passing with confidence, instead of failing with insecurity. Examination questions – together with answers – are furnished as the basic vehicle for study so that the mysteries of the examination and its compounding difficulties may be eliminated or diminished by a sure method.

This book is meant to help you pass your examination provided that you qualify and are serious in your objective.

The entire field is reviewed through the huge store of content information which is succinctly presented through a provocative and challenging approach – the question-and-answer method.

A climate of success is established by furnishing the correct answers at the end of each test.

You soon learn to recognize types of questions, forms of questions, and patterns of questioning. You may even begin to anticipate expected outcomes.

You perceive that many questions are repeated or adapted so that you can gain acute insights, which may enable you to score many sure points.

You learn how to confront new questions, or types of questions, and to attack them confidently and work out the correct answers.

You note objectives and emphases, and recognize pitfalls and dangers, so that you may make positive educational adjustments.

Moreover, you are kept fully informed in relation to new concepts, methods, practices, and directions in the field.

You discover that you are actually taking the examination all the time: you are preparing for the examination by "taking" an examination, not by reading extraneous and/or supererogatory textbooks.

In short, this PASSBOOK®, used directedly, should be an important factor in helping you to pass your test.

CERTIFIED NURSE EXAMINATION SERIES

NURSING EXAMINATION RESOURCES

A variety of tests and programs are available through a number of organizations that will aid and help prepare candidates for nursing certification:

AMERICAN NURSES CREDENTIALING CENTER (ANCC)

The American Nurses Credentialing Center (ANCC) is a subsidiary of the American Nurses' Association (ANA), and the largest nursing credentialing organization in the United States. The ANCC Commission on Certification offers approximately 40 examinations including advanced practice specialties for nurse practitioners and clinical nurse specialists.

Certification is a most important way for you to show that you are among the best in your field – an extra step for you and your career, a step *beyond* state licensing. It gives you recognition and status on a *national* basis.

ANCC certification exams are offered twice a year in May and October in paper-and-pencil format, and throughout the year as computer-based exams. All exams are multiple choice and cover knowledge, understanding and application of professional nursing practice and theory. The time allotted for both the paper-and-pencil and computer certification exams is 3 hours and 30 minutes.

Each exam is developed in cooperation with an individual Content Expert Panel (CEP) composed of experts representing specific areas of certification. These panels analyze the professional skills and abilities required and then define which content should be covered and how strongly emphasized. Test questions are written by certified nurses in their discipline and reviewed by the ANCC to ensure validity and quality.

Exams are scored on a scale, and will be reported as either "Pass" or "Fail." Those who fail the exam will receive diagnostic information for each area of the test. There is a minimum 90-day waiting period from the date of the failed exam for those looking to retake it. For those who pass the exam, a certificate, official identification card and pin will be sent. Certification is valid for five years.

For further information and application for admission to candidacy for certification, write to:
American Nurses Credentialing Center
8515 Georgia Ave., Suite 400
Silver Spring, MD 20910-3492

You can also contact the ANCC and receive further details regarding certification exams and registration by visiting its home on the Internet – www.nursecredentialing.org – or by phone (1-800-284-CERT). Test Content Outlines (TCO) for each exam can also be found on the ANCC website, detailing the format and content breakdown of the test as well as the content areas the examinee should be prepared for.

NATIONAL CERTIFICATION CORPORATION

NCC CERTIFICATION

NCC – the National Certification Corporation for the Obstetric, Gynecologic and Neonatal Nursing specialties – is an independent certification organization. NCC was established in 1975 as a non-profit corporation for the purpose of sponsoring a volunteer certification program.

BENEFITS OF CERTIFICATION

Certification serves as an added credential to attest to attainment of special knowledge beyond the basic nursing degree. Certification serves to maintain and promote quality nursing care by providing a mechanism to nurses to demonstrate their special knowledge in a specific nursing area.

Promotion of quality care through certification benefits not only the individual nurse and the profession of nursing, but the public as well. Certification documents to employers, professional colleagues and health team members that special knowledge has been achieved, provides for expanded career opportunities and advancement within the specialty of OGN nursing, and elevates the standards of the obstetric, gynecologic and neonatal nursing practice.

Certification granted by NCC is pursuant to a voluntary procedure intended solely to test for special knowledge.

NCC does not purport to license, to confer a right or privilege upon, nor otherwise to define qualifications of any person for nursing practice.

The significance of certification in any jurisdiction or institution is the responsibility of the candidate to determine. The candidate should contact the appropriate state board of nursing or institution.

EXAMINATION DEVELOPMENT

NCC selects educators and practitioners in both nursing and medicine who possess expertise in the specialty areas within the obstetric, gynecologic and neonatal nursing and related fields to serve on the test committees. Responsibilities of the test committees include coordination of overall development of certification examinations and development of materials to assist candidates to assess readiness to participate in the certification process.

EXAMINATION DESCRIPTION

Each of the examinations consists of 200 multiple-choice questions. Two forms of each examination are often given to provide the opportunity to perform statistical procedures which ensure added reliability to the total examination process. The examinations are offered only in English and are designed to test special knowledge.

The examinations are given once each in the morning and afternoon, Monday through Friday, at more than 100 test centers. Four hours are allotted for completion of the examination.

THE CERTIFICATION PROCESS

1. Applicants must complete and file a certification application and appropriate documentation and fees
2. An acknowledgment postcard is sent to each applicant when NCC receives the application
3. Eligibility to participate is determined
4. Applicant is notified of eligibility status and eligible candidate receives a Candidate Guide to NCC Certification (4 to 6 weeks from receipt of application)
5. Candidates will schedule their own appointment for an examination time and location, and must take the exam within a 90-day period from notification of eligibility
6. Test administration occurs
7. Examinations are scored and analyzed
8. Candidates receive score reports upon completion of computerized testing (not paper testing)
9. Candidates are notified of certification status, receive information about certification maintenance and are later issued formal certificates

REVIEW COURSES AND NCC

NCC does not sponsor or endorse any review courses or materials for the certification examinations, because to do so would be a conflict of interest.

NCC is not affiliated with and does not provide input or information for any review courses or materials that other organizations may offer.

NCC views certification as an evaluative process. Eligibility criteria have been established to identify a minimum level of preparation for the exams.

CANDIDATE GUIDE TO NCC CERTIFICATION

Each candidate determined eligible to participate in the NCC certification process will be sent a Guide to NCC Certification. These guides can also be found online at the NCC website (www.nccnet.org). The Candidate Guides contain:

- General policies and procedures about the certification process
- Competency Statements that serve as a role description for the specialty nurse
- Expanded examination content outline
- Bibliography of references
- Sample questions to familiarize candidates with examination format (*These questions are not representative of exam content or difficulty level)

The Candidate Guide is not provided as study material, but to assist candidates in evaluating their own nursing practice as they prepare for the certification examination through identification of potential areas of strength and weakness.

SCORING OF EXAMINATIONS

Passing scores are determined based on a criterion-referenced system. Criterion passing scores are established by the NCC Board of Directors in conjunction with the NCC Test Committees using standard psychometric procedures.

Each question is statistically analyzed and evaluated with psychometric consultation, and scores are computed based on this evaluation.

Candidates who take the computerized form of the certification exam will receive their score reports upon completion of the exam. Those who take the paper/pencil exam will not receive their score reports for several weeks after administration.

NOTIFICATION AND AWARDING OF CERTIFICATION

Each candidate is notified of the success or failure to achieve certification. Successful candidates receive a formal certificate and will be able to use the initial RNC (Registered Nurse Certified) to indicate certification status.

Certification is awarded for a period of three years. Initial certification is effective from the date of notification to December 31 of the third full calendar year following notification. Subsequent periods of certification are subject to policies of the Certification Maintenance Program.

CERTIFICATION MAINTENANCE

The NCC Certification Maintenance Program allows the certified nurse to maintain NCC certification status.

Certification status must be maintained on an ongoing basis every three years through demonstration of approved continuing education or reexamination. Certification that is not maintained through the Certification Maintenance Program may only be regained by reexamination.

Specific information about the Certification Maintenance Program is provided to successful certification candidates and may also be obtained by contacting the NCC website (www.nccnet.org).

GENERAL POLICIES

All required practice experience/employment must have occurred while the applicant is/was a U.S. or Canadian RN. Graduate Nurse or Interim Permit status is acceptable, but must be indicated separately on the application form in addition to original licensure information.

NCC defines employment as practice in any of the following settings: direct patient care, educational institutions, administration or research.

When meeting educational requirements, all coursework, including that not directly related to specialty areas, thesis work and/or other program requirements must be completed at the time the application is filed.

It is the policy of NCC that no individual shall be excluded from the opportunity to participate in the NCC certification program on the basis of race, national origin, religion, sex, age or handicap.

All applications received are subject to the nonrefundable application fee ($250 paper/pencil; $300 computer).

Incomplete applications or applications submitted without appropriate fees will be returned and subject to all policies, fees and deadlines.

Applicants determined eligible (whether the candidate has been notified or not) and withdrawn will be subject to stated refund policies.

All NCC policies and requirements are subject to change without notice.

RETEST POLICIES

The NCC does not limit the number of times a candidate may retake the NCC Certification Examinations. Unsuccessful candidates who wish to be retested must reapply, submit all applicable fees and documentation, and re-establish eligibility.

Eligibility: All eligibility criteria of practice experience and/or educational preparation must be met by the time of application. It is the candidate's decision to choose the appropriate examination, based on the content outline, the individual's practice experience and NCC eligibility criteria.

Forms: All required forms must be submitted, and must include all requested information. If the forms are missing information, your application will be returned or you may be found ineligible to sit for the exam. Be sure the RN licensure information is completed. Be sure your documentation is signed by your supervisor or program director, with his/her title indicated, and the date the form is signed. Review your forms before you submit them.

Fees and Refunds: The proper fee must be submitted with your application or it will be returned.

For a current exam catalog containing current fees, terms, filing deadlines and exam dates, contact the NCC at www.nccnet.org, call (312) 951-0207 or fax at (312) 951-9475.

National Certification Corporation
PO Box 11082
Chicago, IL 60611-0082

CENTER FOR CERTIFICATION PREPARATION AND REVIEW

The Center for Certification Preparation and Review (CCPR) provides practice examinations developed by nurses and is intended to familiarize candidates with the content and feel of the real test. The CCPR practice examination identifies content areas of strength and weakness, provides examples of the type and format of questions that will appear on the examination, as well as information on how to focus additional study efforts.

The CCPR program consists of: study strategies, competency statements, content outline, 160-item examination, answer key and sample answer sheet, performance assessment grid, rationales for answers and cited references. Exams are available for inpatient obstetric, maternal newborn, neonatal intensive care and low-risk neonatal nursing, as well as neonatal nurse practitioner and women's health care nurse practitioner.

More information on ordering these practice exams can be found at www.ccprnet.org.

The National Certification Corporation (NCC), a not-for-profit organization that provides a national credentialing program for nurses, physicians and other licensed health care personnel, offers candidate guides for each of the NCC examinations. These candidate guides contain competency statements, detailed test outlines, sample questions, list of book/periodical references and all NCC policies related to the test administration process.

NCC guides are available in the following areas: inpatient obstetric, low-risk neonatal, maternal newborn and neonatal intensive care nursing, as well as neonatal nurse practitioner, telephone nursing practice, women's health care nurse practitioner, electronic fetal monitoring subspecialty examination, and menopause clinician. These guides, in addition to other information regarding testing, NCC publications and links to other organizations, are available online at www.nccnet.org.

RESOURCES FOR PRE-ADMISSION AND ACHIEVEMENT TESTS IN RN AND PN PROGRAMS

The National League for Nursing (NLN) offers a wide variety of examinations designed to aid students looking to further their education in the field of nursing. NLN pre-admission exams are reliable and valid predictors of student success in nursing programs, and NLN achievement tests allow educators to evaluate course or program objectives and to compare student performance to a national sample. The NLN also provides Diagnostic Readiness Tests, Critical Thinking and Comprehensive Nursing Achievement Exams and Acceleration Challenge Exams.

NLN exams can be ordered in paper form or e-mailed directly to you as online tests. The RN program includes tests in: basic nursing care, nursing care of children, maternity and child health nursing, nursing care of adults, psychiatric mental health and pharmacology in clinical nursing, baccalaureate achievement, physical assessment, community health nursing, comprehensive psychiatric nursing, heath and illness, anatomy and physiology, and microbiology.

NLN achievement tests also cover a PN program, which includes exams in: PN fundamentals, maternity infant, child health and adult health nursing, as well as mental health concepts and PN pharmacology.

NLN Pre-NCLEX Readiness Tests serve as practice and review for the NCLEX. Comprehensive Nursing Achievement, Critical Thinking and Diagnostic Readiness Tests are complementary to one another and help students prepare for nursing practice and to pass the NCLEX.

For in-depth information about the types of tests available, ordering, and additional NLN publications, including the NLN test catalog (available for download), visit www.nln.org.

HOW TO TAKE A TEST

You have studied long, hard and conscientiously.

With your official admission card in hand, and your heart pounding, you have been admitted to the examination room.

You note that there are several hundred other applicants in the examination room waiting to take the same test.

They all appear to be equally well prepared.

You know that nothing but your best effort will suffice. The "moment of truth" is at hand: you now have to demonstrate objectively, in writing, your knowledge of content and your understanding of subject matter.

You are fighting the most important battle of your life—to pass and/or score high on an examination which will determine your career and provide the economic basis for your livelihood.

What extra, special things should you know and should you do in taking the examination?

I. YOU MUST PASS AN EXAMINATION

A. WHAT EVERY CANDIDATE SHOULD KNOW
Examination applicants often ask us for help in preparing for the written test. What can I study in advance? What kinds of questions will be asked? How will the test be given? How will the papers be graded?

B. HOW ARE EXAMS DEVELOPED?
Examinations are carefully written by trained technicians who are specialists in the field known as "psychological measurement," in consultation with recognized authorities in the field of work that the test will cover. These experts recommend the subject matter areas or skills to be tested; only those knowledges or skills important to your success on the job are included. The most reliable books and source materials available are used as references. Together, the experts and technicians judge the difficulty level of the questions.
Test technicians know how to phrase questions so that the problem is clearly stated. Their ethics do not permit "trick" or "catch" questions. Questions may have been tried out on sample groups, or subjected to statistical analysis, to determine their usefulness.
Written tests are often used in combination with performance tests, ratings of training and experience, and oral interviews. All of these measures combine to form the best-known means of finding the right person for the right job.

II. HOW TO PASS THE WRITTEN TEST

A. BASIC STEPS

1) Study the announcement

How, then, can you know what subjects to study? Our best answer is: "Learn as much as possible about the class of positions for which you've applied." The exam will test the knowledge, skills and abilities needed to do the work.

Your most valuable source of information about the position you want is the official exam announcement. This announcement lists the training and experience qualifications. Check these standards and apply only if you come reasonably close to meeting them. Many jurisdictions preview the written test in the exam announcement by including a section called "Knowledge and Abilities Required," "Scope of the Examination," or some similar heading. Here you will find out specifically what fields will be tested.

2) Choose appropriate study materials

If the position for which you are applying is technical or advanced, you will read more advanced, specialized material. If you are already familiar with the basic principles of your field, elementary textbooks would waste your time. Concentrate on advanced textbooks and technical periodicals. Think through the concepts and review difficult problems in your field.

These are all general sources. You can get more ideas on your own initiative, following these leads. For example, training manuals and publications of the government agency which employs workers in your field can be useful, particularly for technical and professional positions. A letter or visit to the government department involved may result in more specific study suggestions, and certainly will provide you with a more definite idea of the exact nature of the position you are seeking.

3) Study this book!

III. KINDS OF TESTS

Tests are used for purposes other than measuring knowledge and ability to perform specified duties. For some positions, it is equally important to test ability to make adjustments to new situations or to profit from training. In others, basic mental abilities not dependent on information are essential. Questions which test these things may not appear as pertinent to the duties of the position as those which test for knowledge and information. Yet they are often highly important parts of a fair examination. For very general questions, it is almost impossible to help you direct your study efforts. What we can do is to point out some of the more common of these general abilities needed in public service positions and describe some typical questions.

1) General information

Broad, general information has been found useful for predicting job success in some kinds of work. This is tested in a variety of ways, from vocabulary lists to questions about current events. Basic background in some field of work, such as sociology or economics, may be sampled in a group of questions. Often these are principles which have become familiar to most persons through exposure rather than through formal training. It is difficult to advise you how to study for these questions; being alert to the world around you is our best suggestion.

2) Verbal ability

An example of an ability needed in many positions is verbal or language ability. Verbal ability is, in brief, the ability to use and understand words. Vocabulary and grammar tests are typical measures of this ability. Reading comprehension or paragraph interpretation questions are common in many kinds of civil service tests. You are given a paragraph of written material and asked to find its central meaning.

IV. KINDS OF QUESTIONS

1. Multiple-choice Questions

Most popular of the short-answer questions is the "multiple choice" or "best answer" question. It can be used, for example, to test for factual knowledge, ability to solve problems or judgment in meeting situations found at work.

A multiple-choice question is normally one of three types:
- It can begin with an incomplete statement followed by several possible endings. You are to find the one ending which best completes the statement, although some of the others may not be entirely wrong.
- It can also be a complete statement in the form of a question which is answered by choosing one of the statements listed.
- It can be in the form of a problem – again you select the best answer.

Here is an example of a multiple-choice question with a discussion which should give you some clues as to the method for choosing the right answer:

When an employee has a complaint about his assignment, the action which will best help him overcome his difficulty is to
    A. discuss his difficulty with his coworkers
    B. take the problem to the head of the organization
    C. take the problem to the person who gave him the assignment
    D. say nothing to anyone about his complaint

In answering this question, you should study each of the choices to find which is best. Consider choice "A" – Certainly an employee may discuss his complaint with fellow employees, but no change or improvement can result, and the complaint remains unresolved. Choice "B" is a poor choice since the head of the organization probably does not know what assignment you have been given, and taking your problem to him is known as "going over the head" of the supervisor. The supervisor, or person who made the assignment, is the person who can clarify it or correct any injustice. Choice "C" is, therefore, correct. To say nothing, as in choice "D," is unwise. Supervisors have and interest in knowing the problems employees are facing, and the employee is seeking a solution to his problem.

2. True/False

3. Matching Questions

Matching an answer from a column of choices within another column.

V. RECORDING YOUR ANSWERS

Computer terminals are used more and more today for many different kinds of exams.

For an examination with very few applicants, you may be told to record your answers in the test booklet itself. Separate answer sheets are much more common. If this separate answer sheet is to be scored by machine – and this is often the case – it is highly important that you mark your answers correctly in order to get credit.

VI. BEFORE THE TEST

YOUR PHYSICAL CONDITION IS IMPORTANT

If you are not well, you can't do your best work on tests. If you are half asleep, you can't do your best either. Here are some tips:

1) Get about the same amount of sleep you usually get. Don't stay up all night before the test, either partying or worrying—DON'T DO IT!
2) If you wear glasses, be sure to wear them when you go to take the test. This goes for hearing aids, too.
3) If you have any physical problems that may keep you from doing your best, be sure to tell the person giving the test. If you are sick or in poor health, you relay cannot do your best on any test. You can always come back and take the test some other time.

Common sense will help you find procedures to follow to get ready for an examination. Too many of us, however, overlook these sensible measures. Indeed, nervousness and fatigue have been found to be the most serious reasons why applicants fail to do their best on civil service tests. Here is a list of reminders:

- Begin your preparation early – Don't wait until the last minute to go scurrying around for books and materials or to find out what the position is all about.
- Prepare continuously – An hour a night for a week is better than an all-night cram session. This has been definitely established. What is more, a night a week for a month will return better dividends than crowding your study into a shorter period of time.
- Locate the place of the exam – You have been sent a notice telling you when and where to report for the examination. If the location is in a different town or otherwise unfamiliar to you, it would be well to inquire the best route and learn something about the building.
- Relax the night before the test – Allow your mind to rest. Do not study at all that night. Plan some mild recreation or diversion; then go to bed early and get a good night's sleep.
- Get up early enough to make a leisurely trip to the place for the test – This way unforeseen events, traffic snarls, unfamiliar buildings, etc. will not upset you.
- Dress comfortably – A written test is not a fashion show. You will be known by number and not by name, so wear something comfortable.
- Leave excess paraphernalia at home – Shopping bags and odd bundles will get in your way. You need bring only the items mentioned in the official notice you received; usually everything you need is provided. Do not bring reference books to the exam. They will only confuse those last minutes and be taken away from you when in the test room.

- Arrive somewhat ahead of time – If because of transportation schedules you must get there very early, bring a newspaper or magazine to take your mind off yourself while waiting.
- Locate the examination room – When you have found the proper room, you will be directed to the seat or part of the room where you will sit. Sometimes you are given a sheet of instructions to read while you are waiting. Do not fill out any forms until you are told to do so; just read them and be prepared.
- Relax and prepare to listen to the instructions
- If you have any physical problem that may keep you from doing your best, be sure to tell the test administrator. If you are sick or in poor health, you really cannot do your best on the exam. You can come back and take the test some other time.

VII. AT THE TEST

The day of the test is here and you have the test booklet in your hand. The temptation to get going is very strong. Caution! There is more to success than knowing the right answers. You must know how to identify your papers and understand variations in the type of short-answer question used in this particular examination. Follow these suggestions for maximum results from your efforts:

1) Cooperate with the monitor

The test administrator has a duty to create a situation in which you can be as much at ease as possible. He will give instructions, tell you when to begin, check to see that you are marking your answer sheet correctly, and so on. He is not there to guard you, although he will see that your competitors do not take unfair advantage. He wants to help you do your best.

2) Listen to all instructions

Don't jump the gun! Wait until you understand all directions. In most civil service tests you get more time than you need to answer the questions. So don't be in a hurry. Read each word of instructions until you clearly understand the meaning. Study the examples, listen to all announcements and follow directions. Ask questions if you do not understand what to do.

3) Identify your papers

Civil service exams are usually identified by number only. You will be assigned a number; you must not put your name on your test papers. Be sure to copy your number correctly. Since more than one exam may be given, copy your exact examination title.

4) Plan your time

Unless you are told that a test is a "speed" or "rate of work" test, speed itself is usually not important. Time enough to answer all the questions will be provided, but this does not mean that you have all day. An overall time limit has been set. Divide the total time (in minutes) by the number of questions to determine the approximate time you have for each question.

5) Do not linger over difficult questions

If you come across a difficult question, mark it with a paper clip (useful to have along) and come back to it when you have been through the booklet. One caution if you do this – be sure to skip a number on your answer sheet as well. Check often to be sure that you have not lost your place and that you are marking in the row numbered the same as the question you are answering.

6) Read the questions

Be sure you know what the question asks! Many capable people are unsuccessful because they failed to read the questions correctly.

7) Answer all questions

Unless you have been instructed that a penalty will be deducted for incorrect answers, it is better to guess than to omit a question.

8) Speed tests

It is often better NOT to guess on speed tests. It has been found that on timed tests people are tempted to spend the last few seconds before time is called in marking answers at random – without even reading them – in the hope of picking up a few extra points. To discourage this practice, the instructions may warn you that your score will be "corrected" for guessing. That is, a penalty will be applied. The incorrect answers will be deducted from the correct ones, or some other penalty formula will be used.

9) Review your answers

If you finish before time is called, go back to the questions you guessed or omitted to give them further thought. Review other answers if you have time.

10) Return your test materials

If you are ready to leave before others have finished or time is called, take ALL your materials to the monitor and leave quietly. Never take any test material with you. The monitor can discover whose papers are not complete, and taking a test booklet may be grounds for disqualification.

VIII. EXAMINATION TECHNIQUES

1) Read the general instructions carefully. These are usually printed on the first page of the exam booklet. As a rule, these instructions refer to the timing of the examination; the fact that you should not start work until the signal and must stop work at a signal, etc. If there are any special instructions, such as a choice of questions to be answered, make sure that you note this instruction carefully.

2) When you are ready to start work on the examination, that is as soon as the signal has been given, read the instructions to each question booklet, underline any key words or phrases, such as least, best, outline, describe and the like. In this way you will tend to answer as requested rather than discover on reviewing your paper that you listed without describing, that you selected the worst choice rather than the best choice, etc.

3) If the examination is of the objective or multiple-choice type – that is, each question will also give a series of possible answers: A, B, C or D, and you are called upon to select the best answer and write the letter next to that answer on your answer paper – it is advisable to start answering each question in turn. There may be anywhere from 50 to 100 such questions in the three or four hours allotted and you can see how much time would be taken if you read through all the questions before beginning to answer any. Furthermore, if you

come across a question or group of questions which you know would be difficult to answer, it would undoubtedly affect your handling of all the other questions.

4) If the examination is of the essay type and contains but a few questions, it is a moot point as to whether you should read all the questions before starting to answer any one. Of course, if you are given a choice – say five out of seven and the like – then it is essential to read all the questions so you can eliminate the two that are most difficult. If, however, you are asked to answer all the questions, there may be danger in trying to answer the easiest one first because you may find that you will spend too much time on it. The best technique is to answer the first question, then proceed to the second, etc.

5) Time your answers. Before the exam begins, write down the time it started, then add the time allowed for the examination and write down the time it must be completed, then divide the time available somewhat as follows:
   - If 3-1/2 hours are allowed, that would be 210 minutes. If you have 80 objective-type questions, that would be an average of 2-1/2 minutes per question. Allow yourself no more than 2 minutes per question, or a total of 160 minutes, which will permit about 50 minutes to review.
   - If for the time allotment of 210 minutes there are 7 essay questions to answer, that would average about 30 minutes a question. Give yourself only 25 minutes per question so that you have about 35 minutes to review.

6) The most important instruction is to read each question and make sure you know what is wanted. The second most important instruction is to time yourself properly so that you answer every question. The third most important instruction is to answer every question. Guess if you have to but include something for each question. Remember that you will receive no credit for a blank and will probably receive some credit if you write something in answer to an essay question. If you guess a letter – say "B" for a multiple-choice question – you may have guessed right. If you leave a blank as an answer to a multiple-choice question, the examiners may respect your feelings but it will not add a point to your score. Some exams may penalize you for wrong answers, so in such cases only, you may not want to guess unless you have some basis for your answer.

7) Suggestions
   a. Objective-type questions
      1. Examine the question booklet for proper sequence of pages and questions
      2. Read all instructions carefully
      3. Skip any question which seems too difficult; return to it after all other questions have been answered
      4. Apportion your time properly; do not spend too much time on any single question or group of questions
      5. Note and underline key words – all, most, fewest, least, best, worst, same, opposite, etc.
      6. Pay particular attention to negatives
      7. Note unusual option, e.g., unduly long, short, complex, different or similar in content to the body of the question
      8. Observe the use of "hedging" words – probably, may, most likely, etc.

9. Make sure that your answer is put next to the same number as the question
10. Do not second-guess unless you have good reason to believe the second answer is definitely more correct
11. Cross out original answer if you decide another answer is more accurate; do not erase until you are ready to hand your paper in
12. Answer all questions; guess unless instructed otherwise
13. Leave time for review

b. Essay questions
1. Read each question carefully
2. Determine exactly what is wanted. Underline key words or phrases.
3. Decide on outline or paragraph answer
4. Include many different points and elements unless asked to develop any one or two points or elements
5. Show impartiality by giving pros and cons unless directed to select one side only
6. Make and write down any assumptions you find necessary to answer the questions
7. Watch your English, grammar, punctuation and choice of words
8. Time your answers; don't crowd material

8) Answering the essay question

Most essay questions can be answered by framing the specific response around several key words or ideas. Here are a few such key words or ideas:

M's: manpower, materials, methods, money, management
P's: purpose, program, policy, plan, procedure, practice, problems, pitfalls, personnel, public relations

a. Six basic steps in handling problems:
1. Preliminary plan and background development
2. Collect information, data and facts
3. Analyze and interpret information, data and facts
4. Analyze and develop solutions as well as make recommendations
5. Prepare report and sell recommendations
6. Install recommendations and follow up effectiveness

b. Pitfalls to avoid
1. Taking things for granted – A statement of the situation does not necessarily imply that each of the elements is necessarily true; for example, a complaint may be invalid and biased so that all that can be taken for granted is that a complaint has been registered
2. Considering only one side of a situation – Wherever possible, indicate several alternatives and then point out the reasons you selected the best one
3. Failing to indicate follow up – Whenever your answer indicates action on your part, make certain that you will take proper follow-up action to see how successful your recommendations, procedures or actions turn out to be
4. Taking too long in answering any single question – Remember to time your answers properly

EXAMINATION SECTION

EXAMINATION SECTION
TEST 1

DIRECTIONS: Each question or incomplete statement is followed by several suggested answers or completions. Select the one that BEST answers the question or completes the statement. *PRINT THE LETTER OF THE CORRECT ANSWER IN THE SPACE AT THE RIGHT.*

1. In evaluating the timing *of* an activity and sequencing the alternatives, a management team at a nursing home should determine the *critical path* through the nursing home's network. The critical path in this context is the element of the activity which

    A. takes the longest to complete
    B. takes the shortest time to complete
    C. requires the most resources
    D. requires the fewest resources

    1._____

2. Which of the following most accurately states the growing trend in the structuring of the nursing home industry?

    A. Greater proportional reliance on public financing
    B. Consolidation into larger health care organizations
    C. Greater reliance on extended-care facilities
    D. Dispersement into smaller community-level facilities

    2._____

3. According to most health care professionals and executives, the most ethically troubling aspects of the Medicaid program is that

    A. recipients must prove their eligibility in accord with the program's provisions
    B. many elderly transfer their assets to children in order to make themselves eligible
    C. taxes from working people are used to provide services to elderly beneficiaries
    D. states are subject to federal regulations in the apportionment of benefits

    3._____

4. Studies of nursing homes have generally indicated that a low percentage of private-pay patients in a nursing facility

    A. is a negative indicator of the quality of care
    B. more typically occurs in urban facilities
    C. usually leads to a greater reliance on physical restraints
    D. may increase the degree to which a facility is subject to federal regulation

    4._____

5. Which of the following payors is/are usually involved in fixed reimbursement programs?
    I. Medicare
    II. Medicaid
    III. Blue Cross
    IV. Commercial third-party insurer

    The CORRECT answer is:

    A. I, II
    B. I, III
    C. II, III, IV
    D. II, IV

    5._____

6. Studies indicate that the MOST common process deficiency in United States nursing homes is

   A. an inadequate care plan
   B. a hazardous environment
   C. unsanitary food
   D. the improper use of restraints

7. The effect of the prospective payment system for Medicare, established in 1983, was to

   A. provide a cost-based approach to reimbursement
   B. establish fixed rates for each Medicare admission by diagnosis
   C. regulate the way in which long-term care institutions competed against each other for market share
   D. establish a new system of organizational review for all health care institutions

8. Most staff experience has shown that the activity with which residents are most likely to need assistance is

   A. eating
   B. dressing
   C. getting in or out of a chair
   D. bathing

9. Federal regulations require nursing facilities to complete minimum data set (MDS) forms for patients within _____ of admission.

   A. 48 hours   B. 14 days   C. 30 days   D. 3 months

10. In most nursing homes, daily life is permeated by a model of staff-resident relationships that is most clearly drawn from

    A. child-care settings
    B. client-centered professions such as law
    C. acute-care medical settings
    D. municipal government and constituents

11. Which of the following were effects of the 1983 introduction of Medicare's Prospective Payment System (PPS)?
    I. Overall decreases in long-term care costs
    II. More flexibility in long-term care reimbursement procedures
    III. More referrals and admissions to nursing facilities
    IV. Early discharge from acute care facilities
    The CORRECT answer is:

    A. I, II   B. II, III   C. III, IV   D. I, IV

12. Nationwide, what is the average total number of nursing care hours per resident day in Medicaid-only facilities?

    A. 1   B. 2   C. 3   D. 4

13. Which of the qualitative techniques for decision analysis attempts to optimize the distribution of scarce resources among competing activities? 13.____

    A. Queuing theory
    B. Regression analysis
    C. Linear programming
    D. Network analysis

14. How many hours of in-service training for nursing assistants is currently required each year by federal regulations? 14.____

    A. 0   B. 12   C. 40   D. 64

15. Which of the following is NOT a trend currently taking place in the demographics of United States health care clients? 15.____

    A. Increasing poverty
    B. A rapidly changing racial and ethnic composition due to immigration and growing minority populations
    C. A trend toward smaller family size
    D. An increase in the percentage of younger clients

16. Which of the following factors are affected by the patient mix at a nursing home? 16.____
    I. Staffing
    II. Service mix
    III. The way in which quality-of-care indicators should be interpreted
    IV. Regulations affecting nursing home activities and staffing

    The CORRECT answer is:

    A. I, II
    B. II, IV
    C. I, II, III
    D. I, III

17. Which of the following is a difference between professional review organizations (PROs) and the older professional standards review organizations (PSROs) established by federal health care regulations? 17.____

    A. PROs are made up of solely not-for-profit, physician-sponsored groups.
    B. PROs are paid by federal grants.
    C. PSROs involve smaller geographic areas.
    D. PSROs were subject to the Freedom of Information Act (FOIA)

18. A nursing home administrator or director of nursing at a nursing home can expect the leading cause of illness or injury among nursing assistants to be 18.____

    A. strains and sprains, mostly involving the back
    B. slips or falls to a lower level
    C. respiratory infection
    D. needlestick injuries

19. The largest association for long-term care facilities in the United States is the 19.____

    A. Group Health Association of America (GHAA)
    B. American Hospital Association (AHA)
    C. Federation of American Hospitals (FAH)
    D. American Health Care Association (AHCA)

20. Of the following aspects of nursing home life, the one most exclusively characteristic of United States facilities is the

    A. housing of residents in shared rooms
    B. degree to which physical and chemical restraints are used
    C. use of geriatric or gerontological nursing staff
    D. attempt to involve family members in formulating a care plan

21. Overall, out-of-pocket contributions from clients now accounts for about _____ % of all expenditures on nursing home care in the United States.

    A. 11 B. 22 C. 33 D. 44

22. Compared to nonprofit nursing homes, for-profit facilities generally tend to

    A. have substantially fewer staff
    B. provide better quality care to Medicaid beneficiaries and self-pay residents
    C. have fewer adverse outcomes from pressure sores
    D. make substantially greater use of physical restraints

23. Which of the following is an element of the bureaucratic model of management?

    A. Interdepartmental collaboration
    B. Positions arranged in a matrix
    C. Generalization of tasks
    D. A consistent system of abstract rules

24. Which of the following is the professional society to which a nursing home executive would belong?

    A. American College of Health Executives (ACHE)
    B. American Health Care Administration (AHCA)
    C. Accrediting Commission on Education for Health Services Administration (ACE-HSA)
    D. American Public Health Administration (APHA)

25. Of the following generalizations about nursing home residents, the CORRECT one is that about

    A. 75% are female
    B. 20% are chairbound
    C. 75% are bladder incontinent
    D. 20% require tube feeding

26. The types of managerial decisions made at organizations such as health care facilities typically include each of the following EXCEPT

    A. programmed-nonprogrammed
    B. inclusive-exclusive
    C. administrative-operational
    D. ends-means

27. Gerontological nurse specialists (GNSs) and geriatric nurse practitioners (GNPs) can improve resident outcomes in nursing facilities by
    I. increasing the ability of a facility to care for more complex and acutely ill patients
    II. reducing the use of hospital services
    III. changing the focus from custodial to rehabilitative care
    IV. reducing the incidence of resident behaviors requiring physical restraint
    The CORRECT answer is:

    A. I, II
    B. II, III
    C. III, IV
    D. I, II, III, IV

27._____

28. Studies indicate that the LEAST common outcome deficiency in United States nursing homes is

    A. poor nutrition
    B. resident abuse
    C. failure to prevent pressure sores
    D. inadequate treatment of incontinence

28._____

29. Nursing homes which make extensive use of urinary catheters should be aware that the practice increases the risk of each of the following undesirable outcomes EXCEPT

    A. abscesses
    B. urinary tract infection
    C. malnutrition
    D. renal failure

29._____

30. Programs for cognitively impaired residents in nursing homes should include
    I. music
    II. space set aside where movements will not disturb others
    III. periods of unstructured activity
    IV. small, confined spaces
    The CORRECT answer is:

    A. I, II
    B. II, III
    C. III, IV
    D. I, IV

30._____

KEY (CORRECT ANSWERS)

1.	A	16.	C
2.	B	17.	C
3.	B	18.	A
4.	A	19.	D
5.	B	20.	B
6.	C	21.	C
7.	B	22.	B
8.	D	23.	D
9.	B	24.	A
10.	C	25.	A
11.	C	26.	B
12.	C	27.	D
13.	C	28.	B
14.	B	29.	C
15.	D	30.	A

TEST 2

DIRECTIONS: Each question or incomplete statement is followed by several suggested answers or completions. Select the one that BEST answers the question or completes the statement. *PRINT THE LETTER OF THE CORRECT ANSWER IN THE SPACE AT THE RIGHT.*

1. Which of the following is NOT a provision of the Omnibus Budget Reconciliation Act of 1987 (OBRA 87)?　　1.____

    A. Nursing homes were encouraged to shift the focus of care from custodial to rehabilitative care.
    B. State Medicaid programs were encouraged to adjust their rates.
    C. Nursing homes were encouraged to develop a resident assessment program for every patient upon discharge.
    D. Nursing homes receiving federal funds were required to ensure a high quality of life in addition to a high quality of care.

2. Which of the following is an element of a *functional* organization, as opposed to a *project* organization?　　2.____

    A. Superior-subordinate boundaries are less clear.
    B. Line functions have direct responsibility for accomplishing objectives.
    C. Prime emphasis is placed on horizontal and diagonal work flow.
    D. Management is a joint venture of many relatively independent organizations.

3. Which of the demographic sectors is most clearly on the increase among nursing home residents?　　3.____

    A. Males
    B. Those over the age of 85
    C. Those with chronic cognitive impairment
    D. Married couples

4. Since 1988, which of the following types of nursing professionals have experienced the smallest percentage increase in nursing homes?　　4.____

    A. Geriatric nurse practitioners
    B. Nursing assistants
    C. Registered nurses
    D. Licensed practical nurses

5. Which of the following is NOT typically a difficulty involved in the use of surrogate decision-makers for cognitively impaired residents?　　5.____

    A. The lack of a formally appointed guardian but several de facto guardians
    B. Illegal or unethical decisions made by a guardian
    C. Difficulty in reversing guardianships once cognitive functions are regained
    D. Difficulty in delineating the scope of decision-making for a guardian

6. Which of the following reasons best explains why many nursing home administrators are reluctant to invest in the training of nursing assistants?   6.____

   A. Extensive use of part-time staff
   B. High turnover rates
   C. Adequate supervision and instruction by supervising nurses
   D. High nursing assistant-to-bed ratio

7. Which of the following management roles pertains to the effort to establish suitable organizational objectives and to implement plans capable of accomplishing them?   7.____

   A. Decisional   B. Strategist
   C. Informational   D. Designer

8. Which of the qualitative techniques for decision analysis derives a mathematical equation to describe or express the relationship between the data of two or more variables over a period of time?   8.____

   A. Queuing theory   B. Regression analysis
   C. Linear programming   D. Network analysis

9. Which of the following is MOST likely to be a characteristic associated with a resident in a nursing facility?   9.____

   A. Receiving psychoactive medications
   B. Physical restraints
   C. Bladder incontinence
   D. Bedfast

10. Which of the following are acceptable means by which the staff at a nursing facility can assure respect for the autonomy of cognitively impaired residents?   10.____
    I. Advance directives
    II. Asking residents for permission before performing any procedure
    III. Surrogate decision makers
    IV. The use of restraints to insure safety
    The CORRECT answer is:

    A. I only   B. II, IV   C. I, III   D. II, III

11. In cases where the use of physical and chemical restraints are an issue for a resident, the course of action is usually dictated by   11.____

    A. the will of the resident's family
    B. the will of the resident
    C. the judgment of the nursing staff
    D. state regulations

12. Which of the following comparisons of fee-for-service (FFS) and managed care (HMO) nursing care is generally TRUE?   12.____

    A. Managed care enrollees are more satisfied with their paperwork requirements.
    B. FFS enrollees are more satisfied with their plan's cost.
    C. Managed care enrollees make greater use of their plan's services.
    D. FFS enrollees are less satisfied with their quality of care.

13. Though advance directives have proven helpful in some cases involving the care of cognitively impaired residents, the practice suffers from the significant difficulty of   13.____

    A. compliance with federal and state regulations
    B. frequent conflicts with the facility's formal care policies
    C. family members who step in after the fact to combat the carrying-out of directives
    D. delineating the areas of decision for which advance directives should have force

14. Each of the following is considered to be an element of the internal management function of a nursing home administrator EXCEPT   14.____

    A. evaluating, training, and developing management personnel
    B. developing and improving management information systems
    C. determining and establishing priorities for new services
    D. defining the general course and goal priorities for the organization

15. The current Medicaid floor for a resident's personal-needs allowance is   15.____

    A. $30 a month   B. $75 a month
    C. $1,000 a year   D. $3,000 a year

16. The 1987 Nursing Home Reform Act provides that nursing assistants must be certified and that they must receive _____ hours of training within the first _____ months of employment in order to be certified.   16.____

    A. 10; 2   B. 40; 2   C. 75; 4   D. 120; 4

17. Approximately what percentage of skilled-nursing facilities in the United States have 24-hour coverage by at least one registered nurse?   17.____

    A. 30   B. 50   C. 70   D. 85

18. The staff at a nursing home has become so overwhelmed with requests for IV feedings that it has to postpone several scheduled sessions. In brainstorming about the possible reasons why feedings could not meet demand, the management team decides to first list all the possible explanations.   18.____
    Which of the following visual tools would best help the team to do this?

    A. Decision tree
    B. Pareto diagram
    C. Payoff table
    D. Ishikawa (fishbone) diagram

19. According to many staff surveys, the main problem associated with the federal nursing home regulations issued by the Omnibus Budget Reconciliation Act of 1987 (OBRA 87) is that   19.____

    A. they focus too much on the rehabilitative aspects of care
    B. the time involved in satisfying documentation requirements detracts from the quality of care
    C. the costs of satisfying staffing requirements decrease the likelihood of profitability
    D. they set an unrealistic standard of care for nursing staff

20. In the 1990s, the type of long-term care facilities which experienced the highest growth rate were

    A. nursing facilities
    B. home care agencies
    C. residential care facilities
    D. adult day care agencies

21. Which of the following is considered an outcome variable involved in nursing home care?

    A. Assessment frequency and completeness
    B. Mortality
    C. Use of restraints
    D. Staffing mix

22. The factor which most clearly distinguishes the long-term care market from the hospital market is the

    A. role of private insurance and Medicare
    B. financial status of the clients who utilize services
    C. demand for services
    D. impact of public welfare on expenditures

23. The *second generation* of federal nursing home regulations, issued during the 1990s, tended to focus primarily on

    A. discriminatory admission practices
    B. resident autonomy and respect for rights
    C. safety
    D. reimbursement

24. The purpose of CON legislation, passed in nearly all states by 1983, was to

    A. regulate the amounts charged by health care facilities
    B. divide professional review organizations into their geographic areas of jurisdiction
    C. provide all nonprofessional and paramedical workers in health care organizations with the same workplace hazard protections as doctors and nurses
    D. force institutional health care providers to obtain state approval for construction or renovation projects beyond a certain cost

25. Which of the following is a likely consequence of the shortage of available nursing home care in many states?

    A. More flexible CON requirements at the state level
    B. Greater selectivity in nursing home admission practices
    C. An increasing focus on the individuals with the greatest need for services
    D. An increase in extended care facilities

KEY (CORRECT ANSWERS)

1. C
2. B
3. B
4. B
5. B

6. B
7. B
8. B
9. C
10. C

11. A
12. A
13. D
14. C
15. A

16. C
17. B
18. D
19. B
20. C

21. B
22. A
23. B
24. D
25. B

EXAMINATION SECTION
TEST 1

DIRECTIONS: Each question or incomplete statement is followed by several suggested answers or completions. Select the one that BEST answers the question or completes the statement. *PRINT THE LETTER OF THE CORRECT ANSWER IN THE SPACE AT THE RIGHT.*

1. The history of the nursing home field, in general, has been tied to   1._____

    A. home health care practitioners
    B. sectarian cooperatives
    C. investor-owned enterprise
    D. not-for-profit public administration

2. Currently, what is the approximate percentage of nursing home admissions that come from hospitals?   2._____

    A. Less than 15
    B. 20-30
    C. 30-45
    D. More than 50

3. The _____ long-term care facility provides on-site registered nursing supervision for one nursing shift per day.   3._____

    A. skilled nursing
    B. intermediate
    C. residential
    D. extended

4. In most traditional models, the quality of nursing home care has been measured by _____ variables.   4._____

    A. structural
    B. financial
    C. procedural
    D. outcome

5. In the 1990s, the type of long-term care facilities which experienced the lowest growth rate were   5._____

    A. nursing facilities
    B. home care agencies
    C. residential care facilities
    D. adult day care agencies

6. The Nursing Home Reform Act of 1987 requires   6._____

    A. at least 12-hour coverage by licensed nursing personnel
    B. at least 12-hour coverage by one or more registered nurses
    C. 24-hour coverage by licensed nursing personnel
    D. 24-hour coverage by one or more registered nurses

7. The input-conversion-output model of health service organizations includes each of the following assumptions EXCEPT   7._____

    A. the organization interacts with, and is affected by, its external environment
    B. the organization is the formal setting in which objectives are accomplished by converting resources

C. managers are the catalysts who cause the conversion of resources into satisfied objectives
D. outputs are obtained from the external environment and inputs go into it

8. Studies indicate that the LEAST common process deficiency occurring in United States nursing homes is

    A. unsanitary environment
    B. improper restraints
    C. a failure to comprehensively assess resident needs
    D. inadequate activities

9. In the past decade or so, the use of gerontological nurse specialists (GNSs) and geriatric nurse practitioners (GNPs) in nursing facilities has generally had each of the following effects EXCEPT

    A. reduced reliance on nursing assistants for direct patient care
    B. improved admission and ongoing patient assessments
    C. reduced use of psychotropic drugs
    D. decreased incontinence

10. In its quarterly scheduling and budgeting meeting, the management team at a nursing home hopes to make an accurate estimate of the time a new activity will require. The team uses the following figures in its estimate: the most optimistic projection is that the activity will take 4 weeks; the most likely time estimate is 6 weeks; and the worst-case projection is that the activity will take 10 weeks.
    According to the standard procedure for making such estimates, the team should figure a period of _____ weeks into its planning and budgeting for this activity.

    A. 4   B. 6 1/3   C. 8 2/3   D. 10

11. The staff at a nursing home has become so overwhelmed with requests for personal meal deliveries that on occasion, some deliveries are not made as scheduled. In brainstorming about the possible explanations why deliveries could not meet demand, the management team decides to survey all relevant staff members and have them rank the reasons in order of importance.
    Which of the following visual tools would best help the team to do this?

    A. Decision grid
    B. Pareto diagram
    C. Payoff table
    D. Ishikawa (fishbone) diagram

12. Which of the following is NOT an attribute that is common to all levels of management in a health care organization such as a nursing home?

    A. Role in formulation of policies which govern the overall philosophy and everyday operations of the organization
    B. Accountability to superiors for results
    C. Formal appointment to a position of authority by the organization
    D. Responsibility for directing work efforts of others

13. Which of the following is LEAST likely to be a characteristic associated with a resident in a nursing facility?

    A. Contactures
    B. Bowel incontinence
    C. Indwelling catheters
    D. Organic psychiatric conditions

14. Which of the following funding sources accounts for about half of expenditures on nursing home care?

    A. Out-of-pocket
    B. Medicaid
    C. Medicare
    D. Private insurance

15. Which of the following projections for nursing home industry is probably NOT accurate?

    A. The expansion of rehabilitative services
    B. A dependence on public and out-of-pocket financing
    C. An increasingly complex case mix
    D. A movement of experienced registered nurses from hospitals to nursing facilities

16. According to the life-cycle model of voluntary inter-organizational relationships, a nursing home in the transition stage would

    A. seek to sustain member commitment
    B. define purposes of the facility
    C. establish professional evaluation procedures
    D. hire or form a management group

17. In the past decade or so, which of the following types of nursing home patients have shown the most obvious growth in number?

    A. The terminally ill
    B. Those who use a nursing facility for recovery and rehabilitation following an acute hospital stay
    C. Those with multiple chronic conditions and cognitive and functional impairments who will remain at the facility for the rest of their lives
    D. Those under the age of 65

18. The _____ long-term care facilities is typically part of a general acute hospital.

    A. skilled nursing
    B. intermediate
    C. residential
    D. extended

19. Which of the following situations or characteristics is most likely to result in a high staff turnover rate at a nursing home?

    A. Inclusion of nursing assistants as part of care team
    B. Provision of free on-site child care
    C. Minimal use of part-time staff
    D. Low nursing assistant (NA)-to-bed ratios

20. Which of the following is considered a process variable involved in nursing home care?

    A. Bladder training
    B. Theft/abuse
    C. Depression
    D. Payor mix

21. Which of the following is a presupposition involved with the use of staffing standards or ratios as an indicator of the quality of care in nursing homes?

    A. Fixed staffing-to-resident ratios can be established across all facilities.
    B. Higher staff ratios lead to improved processes and care outcomes.
    C. Facilities should use case-mix methods for adjusting their staffing levels.
    D. Higher staff ratios will lead to greater revenue due to time-saving measures.

22. In general, which of the following is a process of approving a paramedical employee which involves the appropriate professional association, often in addition to the American Medical Association?

    A. Endorsement B. Licensure
    C. Certification D. Registration

23. Among nursing home residents, the common denominator is

    A. sensory impairment B. functional impairment
    C. cognitive impairment D. involuntary admission

24. Most of the direct care in the nursing home environment is provided by

    A. licensed practical nurses
    B. registered nurses
    C. nursing assistants
    D. geriatric nurse practitioners

25. Since the mid-1980s, which of the following types of nursing professionals have experienced the greatest percentage increase in nursing homes?

    A. Geriatric nurse practitioners
    B. Nursing assistants
    C. Registered nurses
    D. Licensed practical nurses

26. Which of the following funding sources accounts for about 1/10 of expenditures on nursing home care?

    A. Out-of-pocket B. Medicaid
    C. Medicare D. Private insurance

27. The irony of most nursing home policies regarding privacy is that often

    A. the most desirable space in a home is awarded to the least desirable resident
    B. they emphasize the privacy of the staff over that of the residents
    C. the only private space available is dedicated to unpleasant procedures
    D. they are subject to restrictive state CON legislation

28. Which agency of the Department of Health and Human Services is responsible for administering the Medicare and Medicaid programs?

    A. Administration on Aging
    B. Public Health Service
    C. Social Security Administration
    D. Health Care Financing Administration (HCFA)

29. Among all nursing facilities nationwide, what is the average number of nursing care hours provided by registered nurses per resident day? 29.____

    A. 0.5   B. 1   C. 1.5   D. 2

30. Which of the following is a cooperative tactic for negotiating with employees? 30.____

    A. Disclosing only the information necessary to support the organization's position
    B. Maximizing solutions that have joint utility
    C. Stating a problem in terms of the organization's preferred solution
    D. Setting specific goals

KEY (CORRECT ANSWERS)

1.	C	16.	D
2.	D	17.	B
3.	B	18.	D
4.	A	19.	D
5.	A	20.	A
6.	C	21.	B
7.	D	22.	C
8.	D	23.	B
9.	A	24.	C
10.	B	25.	D
11.	B	26.	C
12.	A	27.	A
13.	C	28.	D
14.	B	29.	A
15.	D	30.	B

TEST 2

DIRECTIONS: Each question or incomplete statement is followed by several suggested answers or completions. Select the one that BEST answers the question or completes the statement. *PRINT THE LETTER OF THE CORRECT ANSWER IN THE SPACE AT THE RIGHT.*

1. Which of the following was instituted for the first time by the federal nursing home regulations that were part of the Omnibus Budget Reconciliation Act of 1987 (OBRA 87)?   1.____

    A. The right of cognitively lucid residents to choose their own roommates
    B. Guidelines for the use of physical restraints
    C. Restrictions on resident payor mixes
    D. The right of residents to organize and participate in resident councils

2. Which of the following is an element of classical organizational design rather than more recently formulated approaches?   2.____

    A. Centralized decision-making
    B. High and actively sought performance goals
    C. Open, extensive interaction process
    D. Motivational process taps a broad range of motives through participatory methods

3. So far, advance directives in nursing home care have been used primarily as a mechanism for   3.____

    A. limiting the use of restraints
    B. sustaining a desired level of stimulation and personal attention
    C. limiting life-sustaining treatments
    D. screening out undesirable roommates

4. In the field of health care, the effects of the shift from cost-based reimbursement to rate-based payment have generally included each of the following EXCEPT   4.____

    A. a reduction in the overall types of services and procedures
    B. a reduction in the number of diagnostic and therapeutic procedures
    C. the revision of medical protocols
    D. increased efficiency of operation

5. It is possible, in some instances, for a nursing facility to waive certain federal staffing requirements. In such cases, the facility must obtain a waiver   5.____

    A. at the end of each fiscal quarter
    B. every six months
    C. annually
    D. every two years

6. Nursing homes which make extensive use of tube feedings should be aware that the practice increases the risk of each of the following undesirable outcomes EXCEPT   6.____

    A. lung infection   B. tube misplacement
    C. pain   D. weight loss

7. In recent years, the incidence of injuries and illnesses per 100 workers in nursing and personal care homes in the United States has remained at around

   A. 7   B. 15   C. 26   D. 35

8. Which of the following is generally considered to be a DISADVANTAGE associated with an informal organization?

   A. Restrictive channels of communication
   B. Clashes with the formal organization
   C. The manager's job is made more complex
   D. Destabilizing effect on work groups

9. A formal training program for nursing assistants should always

   A. be limited to functional assessments in order to avoid legal problems
   B. be phased out by the end of the first year of employment
   C. include sensitivity training
   D. be implemented by non-nursing personnel

10. A nursing home director is faced with a 60% probability that the demand for a certain service will increase by 20% next year, and a 40% probability that demand for the service will increase by 10%. The decision is whether to hire another staff member to handle the increased demand, or let the existing staff devise a way to handle the increased demand. Which of the following visual elements might help the director to make this choice?

    A. Ishikawa (fishbone) diagram
    B. Pareto diagram
    C. Nomograph
    D. Decision tree

11. Which of the following factors is currently LEAST likely to affect the demand for nursing home services?

    A. The projected growth of the older population
    B. An increase in the transfer of medical technology to nursing homes
    C. A decrease in the range of services offered
    D. Recent government policy changes

12. An effect of the federal regulations that were issued in 1990 is that state surveys were

    A. redesigned to include financial incentives for quality care
    B. required upon both admission and discharge
    C. required at the end of each fiscal quarter
    D. redesigned to be more outcome-oriented

13. Which of the following is a federal agency with regulatory power over the operations of nursing homes?

    A. American College of Health Executives (ACHE)
    B. Joint Commission on the Accreditation of Health Care Organizations (JCAHO)
    C. Accrediting Commission on Education for Health Services Administration (ACE-HSA)
    D. Health Care Finance Administration (HCFA)

14. Studies indicate that the MOST common outcome deficiency occurring in United States nursing homes is

    A. a failure to maintain the dignity of residents
    B. the inadequate treatment of incontinence
    C. the inadequate treatment of pressure sores
    D. an excessive mortality rate

15. Currently, the most important federal policy affecting the supply of long-term care beds is

    A. social regulations such as those issued by OSHA
    B. state CON legislation
    C. Medicaid reimbursement policy
    D. Medicare reimbursement policy

16. In today's health care market, the main reason most clients prefer subacute care over hospital care is because

    A. the quality of clinical care is much higher
    B. there is a greater emphasis on rehabilitative services
    C. overall costs are much lower
    D. the quality of therapeutic care is much higher

17. Which of the following payers is/are usually involved in cost-based reimbursement programs?
    I. Medicare
    II. Medicaid
    III. Blue Cross
    IV. Commercial third-party insurer
    The CORRECT answer is:

    A. I only   B. I, II   C. II, III   D. III, IV

18. Approximately what percentage of nursing home residents are discharged from a facility within 3 months of admission?

    A. Fewer than 10   B. 15
    C. 35   D. More than 50

19. Recent studies of physical restraints in nursing homes have generally indicated that they
    I. are generally used only when the safety of a resident is threatened
    II. are an effective means of correcting undesirable resident behaviors
    III. tend to increase overall costs to a nursing facility
    IV. are generally overused
    The CORRECT answer is:

    A. I only   B. I, II   C. II, III   D. III, IV

20. In general, nursing home managers who seek to increase the autonomy of residents in their facility should begin by focusing critical attention on the

    A. schedule of activities
    B. staff-resident relationship
    C. amount of space set aside for individual privacy
    D. means by which roommates are selected

21. The Omnibus Budget Reconciliation Act of 1987 (OBRA 87) provided each of the following as a federal requirement of nursing homes EXCEPT

    A. a director of nursing who is a registered nurse
    B. a registered nurse on duty at least 8 hours a day
    C. an administrator who is a registered nurse
    D. licensed nurses on duty 24 hours a day

22. In the nationwide distribution of all health care expenditures, nursing home care accounts for about _____ %.

    A. 7　　　B. 12　　　C. 22　　　D. 41

23. Most federal nursing home regulations, especially those issued more than ten years ago, have focused on

    A. civil rights　　　B. quality of life
    C. safety　　　D. the reimbursement process

24. Which of the following is NOT a generalized trend among nursing assistants employed in United States nursing homes?

    A. About three-fourths have not completed high school
    B. About two-thirds are women
    C. They often come from low-income families
    D. Less than half have any employer-based health insurance coverage

25. Currently, the turnover rate among directors of nursing at United States nursing facilities is about _____ %.

    A. 5　　　B. 15　　　C. 35　　　D. 55

26. Which of the following is NOT generally considered a component of the controlling function in health care organizations?

    A. Developing and improving accounting and budgeting practices
    B. Containing costs of professional services to patients
    C. Motivating, advising, and counseling management personnel
    D. Improving the accessibility of patient care services

27. Which of the following is most likely to be ranked as the top priority among nursing home residents?

    A. Ability to leave the facility for outings
    B. Roommates
    C. Quality of care
    D. Food

28. The management team at a nursing home is at a point in the development of its operations that stakeholders are beginning to receive benefits from their previous investments. According to the life-cycle model of interorganizational relationships, this facility is in the _____ stage.

    A. emergence　　　B. transition
    C. critical crossroads　　　D. maturity

29. Which of the following is considered a structural variable involved in nursing home care? 29.____

   A. Sanitation
   B. Urinary incontinence
   C. Patient satisfaction
   D. Accreditation

30. According to the life-cycle model of voluntary interorganizational relationships, a nursing 30.____
    home in the maturity stage would

   A. seek to motivate employees to achieve the purposes of the facility
   B. manage decisions about the future of the facility
   C. develop criteria for admission
   D. establish mechanisms for coordination and control

KEY (CORRECT ANSWERS)

1.	D	16.	C
2.	A	17.	C
3.	C	18.	D
4.	A	19.	D
5.	C	20.	B
6.	D	21.	C
7.	B	22.	A
8.	B	23.	C
9.	C	24.	B
10.	D	25.	C
11.	C	26.	C
12.	D	27.	A
13.	D	28.	C
14.	A	29.	D
15.	B	30.	B

EXAMINATION SECTION
TEST 1

DIRECTIONS: Each question or incomplete statement is followed by several suggested answers or completions. Select the one that BEST answers the question or completes the statement. *PRINT THE LETTER OF THE CORRECT ANSWER IN THE SPACE AT THE RIGHT.*

1. The general principles a nurse should follow to aid in the prevention of destructive outbursts in elderly people include all of the following EXCEPT   1.____

    A. discussing with the patient factors that stimulate hostility or aggression and giving argument to resolve conflicts
    B. never threatening, scolding, punishing, or shaming the person
    C. redirecting troublesome behavior into constructive channels
    D. quietly giving short, simple, direct responses to prevent additional confusion

2. Depression may alter patterns and styles of daily living. Depression generally does NOT cause   2.____

    A. erratic sleeping patterns varying from insomnia to excessive sleep
    B. a decrease in somatic complaints
    C. withdrawal from friends, family, and environment
    D. talk of suicide or suicide attempts

3. Short-term memory has a small capacity and is useful for almost instantaneous recollection.   3.____
   Factors that increase the risk of short-term memory loss include all of the following EXCEPT

    A. shortened sensory overload
    B. CNS or circulatory deficits
    C. poor nutritional status
    D. hearing losses and visual deficits

4. Early in short-term memory loss, older persons may engage in behavior to cover for memory losses.   4.____
   Later manifestations of more severe memory loss in elderly persons include

    A. failure to recognize when clothing is soiled, forgetting to bathe, wearing clothing longer than has been normal for them
    B. forgetting to prepare food or to eat
    C. forgetting to take medications according to regimen
    D. all of the above

5. Some older people create difficulties in daily living, not only for themselves, but also for all those around them.   5.____
   All of the following are guidelines that caregivers and family members can use in dealing with these negative individuals EXCEPT:

    A. Set realistic goals with the person and be constructive
    B. Do not get the person involved in doing an activity

C. Accept the deprecating, complaining behavior, but continue to recognize positive contributions and outcomes, even as the person negates them
D. Agree on an approach in which all staff members and family members will behave consistently in responding to specified behavior

6. Nursing management of loneliness should never take a shotgun approach. Any intervention needs to be based on a validated diagnosis of the presence of loneliness plus the individual's

   A. times of greatest discomfort or risk
   B. goals for human intimacy
   C. current coping behavior
   D. all of the above

6.___

7. Diagnostic criteria for alcohol abuse does NOT include

   A. alcohol needed when an extra amount of work, besides the normal daily activities, needs to be done
   B. inability to cut down or stop drinking
   C. amnestic periods for events occurring while intoxicated
   D. continuation of drinking despite a serious physical disorder that the individual knows is exacerbated by alcohol use

7.___

8. Alcoholism in the elderly contributes to skeletal defects by causing

   A. osteoporosis
   B. risk of fractures through trauma
   C. both of the above
   D. none of the above

8.___

9. There are several conditions occurring in the central nervous system that are closely associated with long-term alcohol abuse.
   These include all of the following EXCEPT

   A. cerebellar degeneration   B. amyotropic lateral sclerosis
   C. central pontine myelinolysis   D. pallegra

9.___

10. Regarding common drugs and their interactions with alcohol, the use of _____ increases the risk of hypotension.

    A. nitroglycerin   B. monoamine oxidase
    C. both of the above   D. none of the above

10.___

11. Cancer of the colon and rectum are found most often in the elderly.
    Changes in bowel habits and character of stool require the older person to be a good observer and historian, as well as one who can remember other coexisting factors, including

    A. amount of water and other fluids taken during the time period
    B. types of food eaten, for example, fatty foods, no protein, high proteins, or only carbohydrates
    C. changes in activities and exercise patterns
    D. all of the above

11.___

12. In cancer detection approaches in the elderly, _____ may be used to detect cancer of the breast.

    A. breast self-examination
    B. mammography
    C. both of the above
    D. none of the above

13. Some elderly persons temporarily or permanently lose their full ability to masticate, to move the food bolus to the posterior pharynx, or to swallow the bolus to a patent esophagus, stomach, and intestinal tract. Treatment factors that cause such dysfunctions include all of the following EXCEPT

    A. untreated malignancy or metastatic disease of the oropharynx, larynx, esophagus, or gastrointestinal tract
    B. implanted dentures
    C. trismus as a sequel to radiation, edema, or infection
    D. implanted iridium needles in the tongue or floor of the mouth

14. After exposure to an accumulation of 5,000 rads or a total body exposure of 1,000 rads, changes in composition and consistency of saliva occur and it becomes ropy and tenacious.
    These changes provide a positive environment for infection by

    A. candidiasis
    B. herpes simplex infection
    C. both of the above
    D. none of the above

15. Of the following people, those at LEAST risk for managing their daily nutrition in the face of pain and dysphagia are those who

    A. were previously malnourished as a consequence of alcoholism
    B. are taking excessive analgesics
    C. maintained poor oral hygiene prior to, during, and after delivery
    D. have a solitary lifestyle with few personal support symptoms

16. Nursing strategies useful in managing difficulties in eating include all of the following EXCEPT

    A. no analgesia prior to eating
    B. oral hygiene to remove debris, plaque, and tenacious secretions
    C. use of deglutition spoon or modified syringe for liquid diets
    D. considering the option of enteral feeding or hyperalimentation

17. A nurse evaluating the patients response to living each day with the inability to eat should collect data on the status of

    A. oropharyngeal tissues
    B. gingiva and the ability to wear dentures or partials
    C. eating and swallowing skills
    D. all of the above

18. In the over-70 age group, even uncomplicated and successful surgery for cancer results in prolonged low energy levels for almost a year. Certain factors can be predicted to produce periods of low energy.
    Of the following, the factor that does NOT produce low energy is

    A. presence of other decompensating chronic disease
    B. early stages of metastatic disease
    C. neoplastic diseases in which fatigue is an initial and ongoing feature
    D. insomnia or sleep interruptions

18.___

19. Emotional components that contribute to low energy in elderly persons with cancer include all of the following EXCEPT

    A. feeling abandoned by the family or health care providers
    B. pleasant interpersonal relationships
    C. tasks demanding prolonged activity or concentration
    D. social events

19.___

20. All of the following conditions or situations decrease the ability to tolerate pain EXCEPT

    A. presence of gastrointestinal symptoms, for example, nausea, vomiting, diarrhea, constipation, impactions
    B. constant weight loss or cachexia
    C. excessive sleep
    D. emotional upset, such as anxiety, depression, fear, and anger

20.___

21. The factors in cancer and its treatment that increase vulnerability to infection do NOT include

    A. breakdown of skin and mucosal barriers due to tumor mass or treatment modalities
    B. neutropenia and malnutrition
    C. increased phagocytic function of leukocytes
    D. impaired antibody production

21.___

22. The best treatment for infection in older persons with cancer is prevention. The nursing regimen for prevention includes involving the patient and family in all of the following EXCEPT

    A. learning safe handwashing and oral hygiene techniques and patterns
    B. starting with prophylactic antibiotics
    C. learning safe laundry techniques and the importance of changing particular items of clothing and bedding regularly
    D. learning how to clean humidifiers and respirators, oxygen tubing, or other treatment instruments used in daily care

22.___

23. The older person with cancer experiences multiple separations in daily living with the disease and its treatment. Persons well-equipped to handle the separations associated with cancer are those who

    A. feel helpless or hopeless
    B. live alone or have diminishing contact with family and friends, particularly age-mates or favorite people
    C. suffer severe pain or intractable nausea and vomiting
    D. none of the above

23.___

24. Drug treatment can increase the risk of congestive cardiac failure. Inadequate or over-zealous drug therapy can precipitate congestive heart failure.
Drugs with this potential to affect congestive cardiac and heart failure do NOT include

   A. beta-adrenergic blockers
   B. calcium channel blockers
   C. digoxin
   D. alcohol

24.____

25. The most severe complication associated with congestive heart failure is the development of other end-stage organ disease as a result of chronic perfusion reduction.
The goals of treatment that nurses should keep in mind include all of the following EXCEPT

   A. increase cardiac preload
   B. reduce sodium and water retention
   C. improve contractility of heart
   D. reduce cardiac workload

25.____

KEY (CORRECT ANSWERS)

1.	A	11.	D
2.	B	12.	C
3.	A	13.	B
4.	D	14.	C
5.	B	15.	B
6.	D	16.	A
7.	A	17.	D
8.	C	18.	B
9.	B	19.	B
10.	A	20.	C

21. C
22. B
23. D
24. B
25. A

TEST 2

DIRECTIONS: Each question or incomplete statement is followed by several suggested answers or completions. Select the one that BEST answers the question or completes the statement. *PRINT THE LETTER OF THE CORRECT ANSWER IN THE SPACE AT THE RIGHT.*

1. In elderly patients with CHF, methods used to decrease cardiac workload include 1.____

    A. vasodilators to reduce peripheral vascular resistance
    B. weight reduction
    C. both of the above
    D. none of the above

2. Digitalis, a cardiac glycoside, is the standard treatment for increasing the force and velocity of each contraction. Factors that influence the individuals sensitivity to digitalis include 2.____

    A. fluid and electrolyte balance, particularly sodium and potassium
    B. concomitant drug therapies, for example, anti-arrhythmics, catecholamines
    C. altered thyroid or renal function
    D. all of the above

3. While all older persons are at risk for arterial occlusive disease, there are some factors that increase the risk, including all of the following EXCEPT 3.____

    A. being a female
    B. having diabetes mellitus
    C. being a smoker
    D. having a history of coronary artery disease or cerebrovascular disease

4. Complications associated with ischemic heart disease in the elderly do NOT include 4.____

    A. cardiac failure
    B. thyrotoxicosis
    C. cardiac rupture
    D. pulmonary embolism

5. The nursing goals of treatment for older persons with ischemic heart disease include 5.____

    A. increasing myocardial oxygen supply
    B. reducing myocardial oxygen demand
    C. both of the above
    D. none of the above

6. Arterial occlusive disease can range from inconvenience to a severely debilitating disease with serious ischemia and infarction of tissues in the lower extremities. Treatment of arterial occlusive disease in the elderly includes all of the following EXCEPT 6.____

    A. slowing the progression of the disease
    B. increasing collateral circulation
    C. increasing the cardiac afterload
    D. maintaining skin integrity

7. Congestive cardiac failure and other cardiac pathology commonly results in shortness of breath and reduced strength and endurance.
NOT included among the complications in daily living that may occur if it is not managed effectively is

   A. discouragement and depression leading to slow suicide by misuse of medications, sodium consumption, not eating, and self-neglect
   B. excessive sleepiness
   C. malnutrition secondary to anorexia and the inability to shop for or prepare food
   D. use of high sodium convenience food

8. Chronic congestive heart failure and its treatment affect appetite and digestion in several ways.
Factors that increase the problems experienced with food and eating include all of the following EXCEPT

   A. hepatic engorgement and enlarged heart
   B. dyspnea and decreased energy for eating
   C. splenic infarction
   D. persistent electrolyte imbalance

9. Managing eating with the side effects of congestive heart failure can be predicted on the basis of the persons

   A. capacity and eternal resources for purchasing and preparing meals
   B. understanding and acceptance of diet as an important factor in health status and relative well-being
   C. desire to live
   D. all of the above

10. Failure to incorporate appropriate eating into daily living with congestive heart failure can produce a downward spiral in which not eating results in even lessened hunger and leads to all of the following EXCEPT

    A. growing weakness
    B. increasing hepatic and splenic failure
    C. infection
    D. growing cardiac and serum chemistry

11. Prognostic variables on managing daily living with leg pain and intermittent claudication include

    A. rate of progression of the disease and symptoms present
    B. older persons motivation to begin and continue a prescribed exercise program
    C. previous capacity to make adjustments in daily living
    D. all of the above

12. Inability to manage daily living effectively because of leg pain and intermittent claudication in an elderly patient with congestive heart failure will most likely NOT result in

    A. social isolation because of inability to get out
    B. ulceration, gangrene, failure to manage acute emergencies, and resultant amputation or death

C. an angry feeling towards the staff with homicidal ideation
D. malnutrition

13. The nursing regimen in a patient of congestive heart failure with leg pain and intermittent claudication includes planning with the older person or primary care-givers on specific management of daily living as it relates to all of the following EXCEPT

    A. keeping the leg acutely flexed at the hips to enhance circulation
    B. externally supporting leg tissues
    C. planning activities ahead to reduce unnecessary walking in daily chores
    D. planning for alternatives

14. EFFECTIVE management of daily living with symptomatic peripheral vascular disease can be evaluated in terms of the

    A. amount of walking that can be done prior to onset of pain
    B. maintenance of personal care and nutritional status
    C. status of personal feeling of well-being
    D. all of the above

15. In the elderly, leg ulcers heal very slowly, if at all. Deterrents to managing daily living effectively with leg ulcers and their treatment do NOT include

    A. extensive deep, bilateral or infected ulcers
    B. hyperesthesia in legs
    C. lack of assistance in wound care, chores, and transportation
    D. lack of money for supplies and medications

16. Nursing interventions in the management of daily living with leg ulcers include all of the following EXCEPT

    A. teaching dressing, soaking, and wound cleaning techniques as needed
    B. trying to adopt a sitting posture most of the time, keeping the legs down
    C. as debridement is very painful, analgesics can be taken before an office visit
    D. helping the person deal with the reality of the slowness of the healing of ulcers, despite the best of care

17. Certain older persons are at greater risk of managing daily living by not dealing with the signs and symptoms of transient ischemic attacks.
    Of the following, the only people NOT at increased risk are those who

    A. are continuously talking about these minor complaints to the doctor
    B. attribute the signs and symptoms of transient ischemic attacks to aging
    C. have an unclear mental status
    D. are loners with few close associates to recognize changes in their physical and mental states

18. Good prognosis for the effective management of daily living in an elderly patient with transient ischemic attacks includes

    A. being totally preoccupied with the threat and risks of transient ischemic attacks
    B. having a backup support system
    C. having poor skills or an inadequate plan for reporting the symptoms experienced
    D. all of the above

19. Nursing interventions in an elderly patient with transient ischemic attacks addresses several areas of daily living. These interventions include all of the following activities EXCEPT

    A. encouraging or assisting the older person to find a physician or clinician in whom he has confidence
    B. locating the telephone at bedside
    C. encouraging the patient for sudden rapid changes of position and movement
    D. improving the safety of the environment in the home

20. Of the following individuals, those NOT at higher risk for not being able to manage daily living with altered speech and comprehension include those who

    A. live with people or in a community where there is little understanding of the dynamics of pathology
    B. were very non-verbal prior to their stroke
    C. go out in a community where their condition is not recognized or understood
    D. lack a consistent companion

21. A person who recovers from a major stroke faces a long rehabilitation period. Rationale for use of the evaluation flow sheet includes the desire to

    A. assess improvements of functions
    B. enhance self-esteem and body image
    C. recall how much progress has been made since the onset of disability
    D. all of the above

22. The cornerstone of treatment of diabetes mellitus is diet.
    The goal of diet treatment includes all of the following EXCEPT

    A. achievement and maintenance of ideal body weight
    B. taking concentrated carbohydrates
    C. avoidance of wide swings of blood pressure
    D. normal blood fats

23. Factors responsible for symptomatology of hypoglycemia in an elderly patient with diabetes mellitus include

    A. decreased glucose available to brain
    B. epinephrine release with a sympathetic nervous system response
    C. both of the above
    D. none of the above

24. Guidelines for the diabetic patient or for people responsible for the diabetic patient include:

    A. Inspecting feet daily for blisters, breaks, calluses, and bruises
    B. Washing with mild soap and then soaking in water for 15 minutes
    C. Avoiding stockings with holes or mended places
    D. All of the above

25. Helping an older person cope with diabetes is a complex situation. A realistic look at the elderly person seems to justify adjustment of all of the following goals EXCEPT

    A. attainment and maintenance of ideal body weight
    B. presence of hypoglycemia
    C. absence of acidosis and ketonuria
    D. absence of atrophy or scarring of hypertrophy at injection sites

25.____

KEY (CORRECT ANSWERS)

1. C	11. D
2. D	12. C
3. A	13. A
4. B	14. D
5. C	15. B
6. C	16. B
7. B	17. A
8. C	18. B
9. D	19. C
10. B	20. B

21. D
22. B
23. C
24. D
25. B

EXAMINATION SECTION
TEST 1

DIRECTIONS: Each question or incomplete statement is followed by several suggested answers or completions. Select the one that BEST answers the question or completes the statement. *PRINT THE LETTER OF THE CORRECT ANSWER IN THE SPACE AT THE RIGHT.*

1. When developing a conceptual framework for nursing practice with the elderly, a nurse should resolve the question: What

    A. assumptions, beliefs, and values about nursing and the elderly influence my practice?
    B. is the range of expected health outcomes for older persons?
    C. is the nature of the professional nurse's relationship with other health care providers of the elderly?
    D. all of the above

2. Much of gerontological nursing is application of nursing processes and methods, with special attention to the unique influences of the aging process on health and illness. Modifications in elements of nursing practice because patients are of advanced age include all of the following EXCEPT

    A. fast pace of nursing process
    B. attention to the effects of the aging process on disease presentation and responses to disease and treatment
    C. increased alertness for signs of an intensified stress state
    D. financial resources available to implement plan of care

3. Dryness, wrinkling, laxity, uneven pigmentation, and a variety of proliferative lesions of the skin are due to normal aging, the genetic makeup of the individual, and environmental factors, such as sun exposure.
Lichenification is classified as nonpathologic skin lesions found in the elderly and characterized by

    A. well-circumscribed areas of cutaneous thickening and hardening
    B. results from repeated rubbing or scratching
    C. both of the above
    D. none of the above

4. An estimated 40% of Americans 65-74 years of age suffer from a skin disease that is severe enough for them to seek treatment.
All of the following are common pathological skin lesions found in the elderly EXCEPT

    A. psoriasis
    B. seborrheic keratoses
    C. herpes zoster
    D. bullous pemphigoid

5. The incidence of potentially blinding diseases increases dramatically after the age of 65. The one of the following that is NOT among the leading causes of blindness in elderly people is

    A. senile macular degeneration
    B. senile angioma (cherry spot)
    C. senile cataract
    D. acute angle closure glaucoma

6. Breast cancer is the most common malignancy found in women and accounts for 2% of deaths in women over 75 years of age.
   The BEST diagnostic procedure for breast screening in a woman over 50 years of age includes

   A. breast self-examination
   B. annual professional examination
   C. mammogram
   D. all of the above

7. The aging gut may be characterized by decreased secretions, absorption, and motility.
   Of the following, the LEAST likely cause of severe abdominal pain is

   A. gallbladder disease, secondary to inflammation, obstruction, or cancer
   B. acute pancreatitis
   C. torsion of testis
   D. mesenteric thrombosis, infarction, or hemorrhage

8. The prevalence of colorectal cancer increases at 40-50 years of age, doubles every 10 years thereafter, and peaks at 75-80 years.
   Besides colorectal cancer, other causes of blood in stool includes

   A. hemorrhoids
   B. fissures
   C. vascular ectasias
   D. all of the above

9. Within the field of geriatrics, there is an unusually-high probability that nurses will function in a multi-disciplinary approach in providing health care to patients, families and groups of elderly persons. Nurses who work in situations in which they must assume multidisciplinary functions need to

   A. be well-grounded as specialists in geriatrics and gerontology, in the knowledge of normal aging and in the areas of high-risk health problems among the elderly
   B. be visible to consumers, colleagues, and administrators in their nursing roles
   C. offer consultations and expect consultations and referrals on nursing problems
   D. all of the above

10. Persons at greater risk for adverse drug effects include all of the following EXCEPT those who are

    A. of extremely tall stature
    B. 75 years old or older
    C. receiving an excessive number of medications
    D. having renal dysfunction

11. The pharmacist will focus on the names and kinds of drugs being taken.
    The nurse will look at some different dimensions, including

    A. previous patterns of utilization of medications
    B. attitudes towards medications and their effects, side effects, and allergies
    C. ethnic or religious influences on the treatment of illness and health maintenance
    D. all of the above

12. Barbiturates, benzodiazepines, and miscellaneous sedative and hypnotic agents comprise another group of drugs overused by the elderly.
    Barbiturates are to be avoided in the elderly because of all of the following risks, EXCEPT

    A. high potential for addiction
    B. hallucinations and delusions
    C. paradoxical agitation
    D. sedation and ataxia

13. Drugs such as chlorpromazine, thioridazine, haloperidol, and thiothixene are often overused by the elderly. Their continual use may cause

    A. extra-pyramidal symptoms such as drug-induced Parkinsonism
    B. tardive dyskinesia
    C. both of the above
    D. none of the above

14. Adequate nursing knowledge is one key to effectiveness in managing a medication regimen.
    For each drug, certain data is needed, but it is NOT necessary for the nurse to know

    A. the purpose of the medication, its function, and the disease or condition for which it is prescribed
    B. the generic and brand names of the medication, its color, and the size and shape of dosage form
    C. detailed information about the company who is manufacturing the drug
    D. the route of administration, e.g., by mouth, inhalation, intravenous, etc.

15. Which of the following questions should the nurse be able to answer for a discharging patient regarding the storage of a drug?

    A. Does the medication need to be refrigerated?
    B. Should it always be left in the original container?
    C. Does this medication have an especially short shelf life?
    D. All of the above

16. Professional health care providers, especially those providing nursing or rehabilitative patient care, should be competent enough in the practice of oral health maintenance to do all of the following EXCEPT

    A. perform gastric endoscopy routinely to rule out GI-related causes or bad oral health
    B. assess oral health status
    C. manage oral hygiene
    D. integrate oral health maintenance into patient care plan

17. A major responsibility in direct nursing care is to prevent progressive oral dysfunction syndrome.
    The classic and common example of PODS may be found in the institutionalized stroke patient who, after a year of post-stroke health care, displays all of the following characteristics EXCEPT

A. inability to cleanse mouth adequately caused by loss of motor skills for oral hygiene
B. inadequate control of dental plaque with rampant tooth decay and advanced periodontal disease
C. oral problems that are extremely resistant to drug treatment and keep on deteriorating
D. progressive loss of self-esteem due to poor esthetics and a noticeable offensive odor from the mouth

18. Dentures are not necessarily used to sustain life, although many patients will not eat appropriately or socialize when their teeth are out of their mouths. Common denture problems often managed by nursing intervention do NOT include

    A. mixed-up or lost dentures
    B. maintaining good hygiene of dentures to prevent caries or plaque
    C. ill-fitting dentures
    D. broken or poorly functioning dentures

19. Regarding oral health, the nurse who cares for an older person over a period of time should know the

    A. skills and resources employed to maintain oral health and those being avoided or used ineffectively
    B. patterns in lifestyle that are barriers to oral health, e.g., mouth care, lack of professional care, diet, fluids, and smoking
    C. planning and skills associated with patient's self-care of specific problems, such as protecting damaged or friable oral tissue, dry mouth, bad smell, and so forth
    D. locating resources for professional dental care needs

20. Nurses should routinely evaluate the effectiveness of the oral health practices being performed by persons in their charge.
    When a mouth has been cleansed daily over a period of time, it should have all of the following characteristics EXCEPT

    A. dental plaque should not be apparent on teeth
    B. tissues should be extremely smooth around the teeth
    C. patient should appreciate the feeling of a clean mouth
    D. there should be no bleeding when brushing or flossing

21. When dental personnel enter an institutional situation, they should

    A. write all findings, plans, and notes in the chart, with oral hygiene measures specifically written
    B. assist in the training and assessment of oral health maintenance
    C. both of the above
    D. none of the above

22. Each patient needs his own toothbrush, either hand or electric.
    A nurse should NOT recommend a toothbrush with

    A. curved handle and brushing surfaces
    B. soft nylon bristles
    C. bristle part small enough to reach all areas of mouth easily

D. straight handle and flat brushing surface

23. Recommended care of a toothbrush involves all of the following points EXCEPT: 23.____
    A. Rinse the toothbrush with clean, cold water, and use it to remove any retained food and toothpaste
    B. Store the toothbrush in a dark, airtight place
    C. Use an empty water glass or toothbrush holder to store the toothbrush
    D. Replace the toothbrush when the bristles become loose, bent, broken, or worn

24. Electric toothbrushes may be as effective as hand toothbrushes in maintaining cleanliness of the mouth.   24.____
    The recommended method of toothbrushing with an electric toothbrush is to
    A. wet the bristles of the toothbrush with water and place a small amount of dentifrice on them
    B. hold the bristles of the brush lightly against the side of the teeth so that both the teeth and gums are cleaned
    C. brush the tongue side as well as the cheek side of the teeth
    D. all of the above

KEY (CORRECT ANSWERS)

1.	D	11.	D
2.	A	12.	B
3.	C	13.	C
4.	B	14.	C
5.	B	15.	D
6.	D	16.	A
7.	C	17.	C
8.	D	18.	B
9.	D	19.	D
10.	A	20.	B

21. B
22. C
23. A
24. B
25. D

TEST 2

DIRECTIONS: Each question or incomplete statement is followed by several suggested answers or completions. Select the one that BEST answers the question or completes the statement. *PRINT THE LETTER OF THE CORRECT ANSWER IN THE SPACE AT THE RIGHT.*

1. Old people are susceptible to many of the diseases of younger adults.
   Studies of pattern of disease in the United States reveals that the major categories of diseases in elderly people require that special considerations include diseases

   A. that occur to varying degrees in all aged persons, such as atherosclerosis or cataracts
   B. with increased incidence in those of advanced age but not occurring universally, e.g., neoplastic disease, diabetes mellitus, and some dementing disorders
   C. that have more serious consequences in the elderly because of their reduced ability to maintain homeostasis, for example pneumonia, influenza, and trauma
   D. all of the above

2. A screening profile of individuals at high risk for family mediated abuse or neglect includes all of the following elders EXCEPT those who

   A. live at home and whose needs exceed or soon will exceed their families' ability to meet them
   B. have primary caretakers who are expressing interest and sympathy in dealing with care needs
   C. live in families with a norm of family violence
   D. abuse drugs or alcohol or live with family members who abuse drugs or alcohol or have episodes of loss of control

3. Constipation is known to occur in at least 25% of older patients, and many reasons have been cited as potentially influential.
   NOT included among the factors believed to be contributory is

   A. increase in fluid intake
   B. lack of fiber in the diet to stimulate peristalsis
   C. blunting or loss of the defecation reflex as a consequence of neglect of the urge to defecate
   D. lack of exercise

4. Oral health maintenance implies that the nurse provide

   A. daily oral hygiene as part of the total patient nursing care
   B. assessment of the mouth at intervals of time appropriate to the patient's health status and his ability to care for himself
   C. advocacy linkage to dental care when problems are detected
   D. all of the above

5. For millions of Americans over age 65, osteoporosis is a debilitating disease that reduces their mobility and independence.
   Factors thought to increase net bone losses of calcium include all of the following EXCEPT

A. inadequate dietary intake of calcium and vitamin D
B. smoking and excessive alcohol and caffeine consumption
C. excessive physical activity
D. excessive dietary intake of phosphorus and proteins

6. Foods and fluids that aid in the prevention and management of constipation include 6.____

   A. raw vegetables and fruits
   B. at least 6 glasses of water per day
   C. whole grain cereal products
   D. all of the above

7. Suggested treatment and treatment combinations in a woman with post-menopausal osteoporosis include all of the following EXCEPT 7.____

   A. discourage exercise and advise complete bed rest
   B. assure an adequate supply of calcium and vitamin D plus sunlight exposure
   C. take anabolic steroids and estrogen/progestrin combinations as directed by physician
   D. supplement fluoride, especially in areas where water sources are low

8. The physiological, psychological, social, and economic changes that occur in aging people may result in a pattern of living which causes malnutrition and further physical and mental deterioration! for example, they 8.____

   A. cannot afford to do so
   B. have limited mobility which may impair their capacity to shop and cook for themselves
   C. have feelings of rejection and loneliness which obliterate the incentive necessary to prepare and eat a meal alone
   D. all of the above

9. If effective learning is to take place, the instructor must stimulate an interest in the subject of nutrition. It is NOT advisable for a person eating alone to 9.____

   A. set an attractive table, i.e., make meals an event
   B. never watch TV or listen to the radio while eating
   C. eat outdoors when the weather allows
   D. invite guests often for a potluck or meal exchange

10. Special facets of the federally supported nutrition demonstrating-research projects are basic to the success that many of these projects have appreciated. 10.____
    Among the supplemental provisions are

    A. auxiliary services, such as transportation, dental care, and counseling on individual dietary requirements to make it possible for older people to use services
    B. social settings designated for personal adjustment and adequacy of diet
    C. settings conducive to eating meals with others
    D. all of the above

11. Not all primary caregivers experience difficulties in their daily living associated with providing care to the elderly, dependent relatives in their families. Factors increasing the risk of problems in daily living include all of the following EXCEPT 11.____

A. lack of community resources
B. adequate income
C. environmental barriers, such as transportation and housing
D. substance abuse

12. When the demands on primary caregivers and other family members are seen to exceed their resources and disrupt their daily living, emotional responses normally occur. The nurse's role is to help family members

   A. recognize and accept their emotional responses to the situation
   B. accept their responses as abnormal and illegitimate
   C. both of the above
   D. none of the above

13. Restoration or maintenance of balance in a family may require an interdisciplinary team. It becomes important that one member of that team be identified as the coordinator responsible for the case management.
This individual has a responsibility to

   A. coordinate services and conduct case conferences
   B. keep team members informed about the care plans
   C. conduct ongoing evaluations and updates of the evaluation plans
   D. all of the above

14. Delirium is a common condition, particularly in the hospital setting, and is most often a manifestation of serious systemic disease or an abnormal response to treatment. Diagnostic criteria of delirium includes all of the following EXCEPT

   A. clouding of consciousness
   B. loss of intellectual abilities of sufficient severity to interfere with social or occupational functioning
   C. clinical features that develop over a short period of time and tend to fluctuate over the course of the day
   D. disorientation and memory impairment

15. Dementias are actually a group of diseases sharing a gradual onset, global decline in intellectual capacity and performance, and progressive social incapacitation. The one of the following that is NOT a type of primary dementia is

   A. primary degenerative dementia (Alzheimer's disease)
   B. multi-infarct dementia
   C. Parkinson's dementia
   D. Pick's disease

16. Dementia is an ancient term taken from Latin and literally means *out of one's mind.* Diagnostic criteria for dementia include all of the following EXCEPT

   A. loss of intellectual abilities of sufficient severity to interfere with social or occupational functioning
   B. clouding of consciousness
   C. memory impairment
   D. impaired judgment

17. Nurses may feel some diagnostic confusion between delirium and dementia. Of the following, the feature that favors the diagnosis of dementia is:

    A. Onset of disease is rapid and duration of disease is hours to weeks
    B. Awareness is always impaired
    C. Course of disease is relatively stable
    D. Physical illness or drug toxicity is usually present

18. An older man is on MAO inhibitors for depressive disorder. The nurse should restrict all of the following foods to avoid hypertensive disorder EXCEPT

    A. old cheese
    B. chocolate
    C. white meat
    D. red wines

19. Agitation and restlessness are two of the most pressing behavioral problems that create difficulties in managing everyday living.
    Deterioration is LEAST likely to occur

    A. during periods of fatigue
    B. during early morning hours
    C. following ingestion of certain medications, e.g., indomethacin, pentazocin, and phenytoin, etc.
    D. when infections are present

20. Daily living is MOST likely to be compromised in the presence of agitation and restlessness when those around the agitated person

    A. cannot tolerate the behavior
    B. understand the phenomenon
    C. have workable strategies for dealing with situations
    D. all of the above

21. Manifestations of agitation and restlessness are wide-ranging in both form and severity, including all of the following EXCEPT

    A. long attention span
    B. constantly moving hands, e.g., picking at clothing, dressing and undressing, hand wringing, and twisting paper
    C. an inability to sit still, even for meals
    D. prowling aimlessly about neighborhood

22. Evidences that the everyday living of these agitated and restless elderly persons is not being managed effectively include

    A. exhaustion from lack of sleep or rest
    B. weight loss from burning more calories than they take time to eat
    C. being abused, assaulted, or robbed
    D. all of the above

23. Of the following, which is NOT a goal of nursing treatment plans for restless and agitated persons?

    A. Maintaining nutrition and elimination
    B. Arranging for adequate sleep and rest
    C. Providing a safe, completely isolated environment
    D. Providing for a more comfortable lifestyle

24. Older persons who are MORE likely to manage their current daily living by engaging in aggressive, hostile, and combative behavior are usually

    A. experiencing hearing or vision losses
    B. sharing living space with a person who has similar sensory deficits
    C. frustrated with self at being unable to do what was formerly possible
    D. all of the above

25. Factors that predict the likelihood of hostile, combative behavior continuing as an element in daily living include all of the following EXCEPT

    A. previous pattern of episodes of this behavior
    B. evidence of such behavior in the family
    C. nature of the events that triggers the behavior and the likelihood that such events will recur
    D. the nature of reinforcement the behavior has received

KEY (CORRECT ANSWERS)

1. D	11. B
2. B	12. A
3. A	13. D
4. D	14. B
5. C	15. C
6. D	16. B
7. A	17. C
8. D	18. C
9. B	19. B
10. D	20. A

21. A
22. D
23. C
24. D
25. B

EXAMINATION SECTION
TEST 1

DIRECTIONS: Each question or incomplete statement is followed by several suggested answers or completions. Select the one that BEST answers the question or completes the statement. *PRINT THE LETTER OF THE CORRECT ANSWER IN THE SPACE AT THE RIGHT.*

1. Substance abuse is a major health care problem in the United States. 1.____
   All of the following statements regarding geriatric consideration in substance abuse are accurate EXCEPT:

   A. Most elderly people are taking sedatives which, when combined with alcohol, can be dangerous
   B. Response to treatment is lowest for this age group
   C. 70% of all hospitalized older persons and up to 50% of nursing home residents have alcohol-related problems
   D. Symptoms may go unnoticed or be attributed to other diseases or as part of the aging process

2. Because of strong physical dependence that develops as a result of alcoholism, withdrawal from alcohol is potentially life-threatening. 2.____
   Among the symptoms of alcohol withdrawal are

   A. increased psychomotor hyperactivity with tremors and insomnia
   B. acute anxiety and hyperalertness
   C. auditory or visual hallucinations
   D. all of the above

3. Nursing intervention in the treatment of impending alcohol withdrawal includes all of the following EXCEPT 3.____

   A. monitoring vital signs every 3 hours and notifying a physician of any abnormal readings
   B. administering lithium carbonate promptly
   C. providing a quiet, non-stimulating environment
   D. allowing a patient to express his fears regarding withdrawal and providing non-judgmental, caring concern

4. Nursing care of a patient with alcohol withdrawal delirium would include 4.____

   A. monitoring vital signs and neurological status hourly
   B. restraining patient to prevent injury if needed
   C. stimulating patient to cough and breathe deeply every 2 hours
   D. all of the above

5. Barbiturate withdrawal occurs 48-72 hours after the last dosage and is potentially fatal. 5.____
   All of the following are signs and symptoms of barbiturate withdrawal EXCEPT

   A. postural hypotension
   B. hypothermia
   C. agitation and grand mal seizures
   D. insomnia and psychosis

6. Nursing care of patients withdrawing from barbiturates would NOT include

   A. frequently re-orienting the patient to reality and person, place, and time
   B. conveying a concerned, caring attitude and giving the patient an opportunity to talk about his fears and feelings regarding withdrawal
   C. providing a stimulating environment to decrease agitation
   D. instituting seizure precautions

7. Of the following, the one which a nurse should NOT do when caring for a patient in an acute phase of cocaine overdose who is showing decreased cardiac output related to reduced stroke volume is

   A. monitor and record vital signs every hour until stable and then every 3 hours
   B. allow caffeinated beverages and food
   C. provide a quiet, non-stimulating environment
   D. administer IV propanolol as ordered

8. Regardless of the health care setting, nurses will encounter a substantial number of patients with substance abuse disorders.
   Psychosocial signs (symptoms) important in the evaluation of a patient with substance abuse include

   A. a history of suicidal attempts and complaints of anxiety or depression
   B. a deterioration in performance at work or school
   C. poor impulse control and financial difficulties, with a history of physical or sexual abuse
   D. all of the above

9. The most common cause of anesthesia-induced death in North America is malignant hyperthermia.
   _____ are among the common signs and symptoms of malignant hyperthermia.

   A. Tachycardia and tachypnea
   B. Cyanosis, fever, and skin mottling
   C. Unstable blood pressure and dysrhythmias
   D. All of the above

10. Primary nursing goals for the immediate post-operative period include all of the following EXCEPT

    A. ensuring patient safety and maintaining an open airway
    B. dissipating residual anesthesia and stabilizing vital signs
    C. providing emotional reassurance and decreasing anxiety
    D. none of the above

11. A multitude of possible problems or complications may be encountered in the post-anesthesia period.
    Hypotension in the post-anesthesia period may be caused by all of the following EXCEPT

    A. excess fluid administration
    B. cutaneous vasodilation with rewarming
    C. loss of sympathetic tone
    D. myocardial dysfunction

12. Nutritional deficiencies are associated with impaired wound healing. The contributions of amino acids in wound healing do NOT include their participation in

    A. neovascularization
    B. lymphocyte formation and fibroblast proliferation
    C. absorption, transport and metabolism of calcium
    D. collagen synthesis

13. In an elderly patient undergoing surgery, intrinsic risk factors associated with the development of post-operative venous thrombosis include all of the following EXCEPT

    A. oral contraceptive use   B. hypocoagulation states
    C. dehydration   D. obesity and malnutrition

14. Paralytic ileus is a condition of diminished or absent paralysis which occurs, to some degree, following all abdominal operations.
    _____ is(are) NOT included among the signs and symptoms of paralytic ileus.

    A. Increased bowel sounds   B. Vomiting
    C. Abdominal distention   D. A feeling of fullness

15. The device most commonly used to monitor the ability to take a deep breath is the *incentive spirometer*. Incentive spirometry is commonly indicated

    A. pre- and post-operatively, especially for thoracic and upper abdominal procedures
    B. when a patient is at risk for or has developed atelactasis
    C. when a history of chronic respiratory disease, neuro-muscular disease, or retained secretion exists
    D. all of the above

16. When an incentive spirometry is to be performed, the nurse educating the patient should NOT advise him to

    A. sit as upright as can be tolerated and seal his lips around the mouthpiece
    B. inhale quickly and not try to hold his breath
    C. remove the mouthpiece from his mouth and breathe out slowly
    D. repeat this process for 10 breaths and cough after the last breath

17. An important role of the nurse is to instruct and assist the patient in producing an effective cough.
    Her advice regarding the ability to cough should include all of the following EXCEPT

    A. pain limits the degree of chest expansion, so effective analgesia should be given before coughing exercises
    B. splinting a painful area during coughing with gentle hand pressure makes coughing easier
    C. supine position is the most effective and comfortable position for coughing exercises
    D. oral hydration using ice chips or sips of water can make coughing easier

18. Postural drainage is accomplished by positioning the patient to promote mucus flow through gravity.
    All of the following contraindicate postural drainage EXCEPT

A. head, neck, chest, or spinal injuries
B. decreased intracranial pressure
C. uncontrolled hypertension
D. pulmonary edema or embolism

19. Therapeutic percussion is typically performed by the nurse, while the patient is in various PD positions, to dislodge mucus from the airways.
Which of the following are contraindications for percussion and vibration?   19.____

   A. Recent epidural spinal infusion
   B. Spinal anesthesia or pacemaker placements
   C. Thoracic skin grafts, burns, infections, or open wounds
   D. All of the above

20. Suctioning is sometimes indicated in older people who are unable to clear their secretions by coughing.
All of the following are common complications of suctioning EXCEPT   20.____

   A. hyper-oxemia
   B. atelactasis
   C. damage to airway epithelium
   D. direct vagal stimulation, which may cause arrhythmias

21. Advanced disease resulting from oxygen toxicity manifests itself in a pneumonia-like picture, showing   21.____

   A. infiltrates of chest x-ray
   B. cyanosis and possibly hemoptysis
   C. pulmonary edema
   D. all of the above

22. Some patients continue oxygen therapy following discharge. _____ do(es) NOT indicate home oxygen therapy.   22.____

   A. Pulmonary hypotension
   B. Recurrent congestive heart failure
   C. Erythrocytosis and impaired cognitive processes
   D. Sleep apnea syndrome

23. *Artificial airways* are devices designed to maintain patent communication between the tracheo-bronchial tree and the air supply in the external environment.
All of the following are indications for endotracheal intubation EXCEPT the   23.____

   A. institution of mechanical ventilation
   B. obstruction of the airway above the level of the epiglottis
   C. patient's inability to clear secretions
   D. delivery of accurate oxygen concentrations

24. Nursing care of a patient with coronary artery disease includes all of the following statements of advice for the avoidance of risk factors to the progression of disease EXCEPT: 24.____

   A. Maintain ideal body weight, appropriate for build, gender, and size
   B. Maintain a regular exercise program three to five times per week

C. Follow a high cholesterol, high sodium diet
D. Practice appropriate methods for relaxation daily

25. Nursing advice for a patient with myocardial infarction would be to avoid activities that may increase the myocardial oxygen demand.
The statement of advice below that the nurse would NOT provide is to

   A. avoid excessive caffeine intake
   B. perform a good amount of physical activities after meals
   C. avoid activities known to cause anginal pain
   D. avoid alcohol or drink alcohol only in moderation

26. Nursing advice regarding the intake of medication in a patient of coronary artery disease would include which of the following:

   A. Do not stop medication, skip dose, or make up forgotten doses without a physician's approval
   B. Report any side effects, changes in anginal symptoms, or undesirable effects to a physician
   C. Take medication as prescribed and avoid over-the-counter medications
   D. All of the above

27. Contraindications for thromolytics in a patient with myocardial infarction include

   A. bleeding disorders like hemophilia or thrombocytopenia
   B. a history of cerebrovascular accidents
   C. severe uncontrolled hypertension
   D. all of the above

28. Expected outcomes for a patient with myocardial infarction include all of the following EXCEPT

   A. relief of chest pain and reduction of anxiety
   B. verbalization of fears, concerns, and questions
   C. inadequate cardiac output
   D. performance of activities of daily living without pain or fatigue

29. The incidence of endocarditis has decreased dramatically over the past 20 years as a result of increased awareness of risk factors, effective antibiotic therapy, and prophylaxis. Nursing goals of a patient with endocarditis include that the patient

   A. maintain a temperature within his normal limits
   B. maintain adequate tissue perfusion
   C. verbalize a feeling of comfort
   D. all of the above

30. *Aortic regurgitation* is a valvular defect in which blood regurgitates backwards into the left ventricle because of an incompetent, leaky aortic valve.
All of the following are among the causes of aortic regurgitation EXCEPT

   A. systemic lupus erythematosus
   B. rheumatic heart disease
   C. Marfan's syndrome
   D. dissecting aortic aneurysm

KEY (CORRECT ANSWERS)

1.	B	16.	B
2.	D	17.	C
3.	B	18.	B
4.	D	19.	D
5.	B	20.	A
6.	C	21.	D
7.	B	22.	A
8.	D	23.	B
9.	D	24.	C
10.	D	25.	B
11.	A	26.	D
12.	C	27.	D
13.	B	28.	C
14.	A	29.	D
15.	D	30.	A

TEST 2

DIRECTIONS: Each question or incomplete statement is followed by several suggested answers or completions. Select the one that BEST answers the question or completes the statement. *PRINT THE LETTER OF THE CORRECT ANSWER IN THE SPACE AT THE RIGHT.*

1. The Schilling test is the definitive test for pernicious anemia.
   In addition, it is useful in the diagnosis of numerous other disorders, including all of the following EXCEPT

   A. hypothyroidism
   B. meningitis
   C. sprue
   D. liver disease

   1.____

2. A large number of elderly people are affected by a vitamin B_{12} deficiency. Older adults frequently attribute signs and symptoms of this deficiency to age and do not seek medical assistance.
   Among the signs and symptoms of a vitamin B_{12} deficiency is(are)

   A. sore and beefy tongue
   B. apathy mixed with irritability
   C. peripheral numbness and tingling
   D. all of the above

   2.____

3. An elderly male in a car accident sustains abdominal injuries.
   Nursing intervention for this patient would NOT include

   A. assisting with the insertion of a nasogastric tube
   B. keeping the patient NPO
   C. palpating the abdomen deeply to assess any internal injury
   D. inserting foley's catheter and measuring for urine output every 15 minutes

   3.____

4. In caring for a patient with suspected musculoskeletal injury, a nurse would do all of the following EXCEPT

   A. observe for signs of fracture: pain, swelling, crepitation, and loss of function
   B. leave the open fracture uncovered to facilitate healing
   C. immobilize any suspected fractures by splinting the joint above and below the injury
   D. perform a neuro-vascular check in the area distal to the fracture

   4.____

5. An elderly pedestrian survives head trauma after striking against a car.
   To assess for any neurological injury, a nurse would perform all of the following tasks EXCEPT

   A. inspect the scalp, head, face, and neck for abrasions, hematomas, and lacerations
   B. observe for signs of decreased intracranial pressure
   C. assess for sensation and motor abilities
   D. assess the level of consciousness

   5.____

6. Diseases that occur in varying degrees in all aging persons do NOT include

   A. cataracts
   B. arteriosclerosis
   C. diabetes mellitus
   D. benign prostatic hypertrophy

   6.____

7. All of the following are diseases that have more serious consequences in the elderly and cause more difficulty in maintaining homeostasis EXCEPT

   A. congestive cardiac failure
   B. pneumonia
   C. influenza
   D. trauma

8. The following statements support the premise that chronic diseases are very common among the elderly.
   The supporting statement which is NOT true is:

   A. 86% of the elderly have at least one chronic disease
   B. 60% of doctor visits among the elderly are due to chronic disease
   C. The elderly account for 60% of hospital cases but only 7% of the population
   D. 99% of nursing home residents have at least one chronic disease

9. Besides the physical aspect, psychological, social, and cultural factors play a crucial role in the aging process. Developmental tasks of the elderly resulting from these changes include

   A. successfully adjusting to retirement and reduced income
   B. maintaining contacts with friends and family members
   C. viewing one's own death as an appropriate outcome of life
   D. all of the above

10. Disease whose incidences tend to increase with advancing age but which do not occur universally include all of the following EXCEPT

    A. neoplastic diseases
    B. meningitis
    C. diabetes mellitus
    D. dementing disorders

11. *Dementia* is defined as the impairment of intellectual function, usually accompanied by memory loss and personality change.
    Nursing should try to institute all of the following safety measures for patients suffering dementia EXCEPT:

    A. Always put the patient in restraints
    B. Keep the side rails up and the bed in a low position
    C. Never leave anything at the bedside that can harm the patient
    D. Check the patient frequently, especially at night

12. Signs and symptoms of abuse and neglect of an elderly person include

    A. signs of malnutrition
    B. poor hygiene and grooming
    C. omission of medication or overmedication
    D. all of the above

13. Effective intervention in a case of elderly abuse or neglect would include all of the following EXCEPT

    A. removing the patient from the setting of the abuse if necessary
    B. keeping the allegation secret between yourself, the patient and the consulting physician
    C. obtaining the patient's consent for treatment
    D. providing for careful follow-up, as the potential for further abuse is high

14. Post-operative complications of a genito-urinary system dysfunction include urinary retention and urinary tract infection.
    _____ is(are) among the predisposing factors to urinary retention.

    A. Anxiety and pain
    B. Lack of privacy
    C. Narcotics and certain anesthetics that diminish a patient's sense of a full bladder
    D. All of the above

15. Dehiscence and evisceration are wound complications that occur following surgery on the gastro-intestinal tract. The predisposing factors to this condition include all of the following EXCEPT

    A. wound infection
    B. a short surgical incision
    C. faulty wound closure
    D. severe abdominal stretching

16. A nurse intervening in a case of wound dehiscence and evisceration would NOT necessarily need to

    A. notify a physician and prepare the patient for surgical closure of the wound
    B. cover protruding intestinal loops with moist normal saline soaks
    C. place the patient in a sitting position
    D. check vital signs and observe for signs of shock

17. In the treatment of cancer, chemotherapy may cause leukopenia.
    An attending nurse in this case should do all of the following EXCEPT

    A. maintain reverse isolation if the white blood count drops below 1000 m/liter
    B. start immediate oxygen therapy
    C. instruct the patient to avoid crowds or persons with known infections
    D. assess for signs of respiratory infection

18. As a result of radiation therapy for malignant disease, skin itching, redness, burning, oozing, and sloughing may occur on the radiation-exposed area.
    A nurse would advise and help the patient to do all of the following EXCEPT

    A. avoid pressure, trauma, and infection to the affected skin
    B. wash the affected area with plain water and pat dry
    C. use medicated solutions, ointments, or powders that contain heavy metals such as zinc oxide
    D. use cornstarch or olive oil to treat the itching, and avoid talcum powders

19. To treat diarrhea occurring as a complication of radiation therapy, a nurse would NOT have to

   A. administer anti-diarrheal drugs as advised
   B. encourage high residue, low-protein foods
   C. monitor electrolytes, particularly sodium, potassium, and chloride
   D. provide good perineal care

20. Fluid may be introduced into the external auditory canal for cleansing purposes. Appropriate nursing intervention would include doing all of the following EXCEPT

   A. propping the patient up in bed with his head tilted towards the unaffected ear
   B. straightening the ear canal by pulling the auricle upward and backward
   C. inserting the tip of a syringe into the auditory meatous and directing the solution gently upward toward the top of the canal
   D. drying the outer ear with cotton balls

21. Meningitis is most commonly caused by organisms such as meningococcus, pneumococcus, and H. influenza.
A nurse attending to a case of meningitis would NOT be expected to

   A. administer large doses of antibiotics IV as ordered
   B. provide nursing care for decreased intra-cranial pressure and hypothermia
   C. provide nursing care for a delirious or unconscious patient as needed
   D. monitor vital signs and perform neuro checks frequently

22. An adult patient is diagnosed with a brain tumor. Nursing intervention in this case would include which of the following?

   A. Monitor vital signs and perform frequent neuro checks.
   B. Provide psychological support to the patient.
   C. Provide supportive care for any neurologic deficit.
   D. All of the above

23. *Parkinsonism* is a progressive disorder involving the degeneration of nerve cells in the basal ganglia.
The general care of the Parkinson patient includes

   A. providing a safe environment
   B. encouraging independence in self-care activities
   C. improving communication abilities and providing psychological support
   D. all of the above

24. Nursing teaching and discharge planning for a patient of Parkinsonism include all of the following EXCEPT the

   A. emphasis on the importance of limiting mobility
   B. appropriate use of prescribed medications and information about their side effects
   C. most effective methods to limit postural deformities
   D. promotion of active participation in self-care activities

25. *Myasthenia gravis* is a neuro-muscular disorder in which there are disturbances in the transmission of impulses from nerves to muscle cells at neuro-muscular junctions.
A nurse assisting a patient who has this disorder would NOT

    A. promote optimal nutrition
    B. assess muscle strength frequently
    C. administer cholinesterase drugs
    D. monitor respiratory status frequently

26. Myasthenia gravis occurring in men in their sixties and seventies produces all of the following signs and symptoms EXCEPT

    A. diplopia and dysphagia
    B. muscle weakness, which increases with rest and decreases with activity
    C. ptosis, mask-like facial expression
    D. weak voice and hoarseness

27. Nursing teaching and discharge planning for a patient of myasthenia gravis would include instruction regarding the

    A. use of prescribed medications, their side effects, and signs of toxicity
    B. importance of planning activities to take advantage of energy peaks and of scheduling frequent rest periods
    C. need to avoid fatigue, stress, and people with upper respiratory infection
    D. all of the above

28. General rehabilitative care of a patient following a spinal cord injury should provide

    A. psychological support
    B. sexual counseling
    C. the initiation of physical therapy and vocational rehabilitation
    D. all of the above

29. *Bell's palsy* is a disorder of the seventh cranial nerve resulting in a loss of the ability to move the muscles on one side of the face.
Signs and symptoms of Bell's palsy include all of the following EXCEPT

    A. the loss of taste over the anterior two-thirds of the tongue on the affected side
    B. complete paralysis of one side of the face
    C. displacement of the mouth towards the affected side and inability to close the eyelid on the unaffected side
    D. pain behind the ear

30. Of the following techniques of post-operative nursing care, a patient with cataracts would NOT receive

    A. assistance with ambulation once fully recovered from anesthesia
    B. the changing of the first dressing after one week in order to prevent infection
    C. prevention of increased intraocular pressure and stress on the suture line
    D. advice: no bending, stooping, or lifting at home and use the eye shield at night

KEY (CORRECT ANSWERS)

1.	B	16.	C
2.	D	17.	B
3.	C	18.	C
4.	B	19.	B
5.	B	20.	A
6.	C	21.	B
7.	A	22.	D
8.	C	23.	D
9.	D	24.	A
10.	B	25.	C
11.	A	26.	B
12.	D	27.	D
13.	B	28.	D
14.	D	29.	C
15.	B	30.	B

EXAMINATION SECTION
TEST 1

DIRECTIONS: Each question or incomplete statement is followed by several suggested answers or completions. Select the one that BEST answers the question or completes the statement. *PRINT THE LETTER OF THE CORRECT ANSWER IN THE SPACE AT THE RIGHT.*

1. Older adults have an increased risk of developing serious infections. 1.____
   All of the following are factors that increase the older adult's susceptibility to infection EXCEPT

   A. decreased protein reserves and decreased serum albumin slow cellular response to tissue injury caused by invading microorganisms
   B. physical changes such as increased mucociliary activity and increased elasticity of bronchiolar musculature
   C. decreased function of the immune system and slowed response to antibiotic therapy
   D. chronic disease and drug therapy that can produce immunosuppression

2. Immunizations as a protective health strategy are as important for adults as they are for children. 2.____
   An adult immunization program does NOT need to require vaccines for

   A. pneumococcal, influenza, and hepatitis B infection
   B. measles, mumps, and rubella
   C. Candida albicans and herpes zoster
   D. tetanus and diphtheria

3. Third space fluid loss occurs when body fluid shifts into a space outside the normal fluid compartments and becomes unavailable to the body, producing a deficit in ECF volume. 3.____
   The one of the following which is NOT a possible cause of third space fluid loss is

   A. peritonitis and ascites
   B. overzealous use of diuretics
   C. fistulous drainage
   D. thrombophelibitis and acute pancreatitis

4. Effective nursing management of a patient with hyponatremia should include all of the following EXCEPT 4.____

   A. monitoring fluid losses and gains by accurate measurement of intake, output, and daily weights
   B. monitoring for changes in the sensorium and other neurological disruptions
   C. strongly discouraging the intake of foods and fluids with high sodium content
   D. checking lungs for crackles' and noting other signs of circulatory overload

5. Signs and symptoms of magnesium deficiency are primarily related to the neuro-muscular system. 5.____
   When nursing a patient with hypomagnesimia, it is NOT necessary to

A. check every 5 minutes or before each dose for flacci-dity and loss of patellar reflexes
B. administer calcium gluconate slowly and with caution
C. be alert for laryngeal stridor and take safety precautions for patients with neuro-muscular symptoms
D. monitor the heart rate and check vital signs at regular intervals

6. Most of the signs and symptoms present in a patient are related to a deficiency of ATP, 2, 3 Diphosphoglycerate, or both.
Nursing management of this case depends on all of the following EXCEPT

   A. monitoring for hemolytic anemia, which may occur because of the fragility of the red blood cells
   B. assessing for signs of hypoxia, such as restlessness, confusion, chest pain, and cyanosis
   C. intravenous administration of calcium
   D. monitoring respiratory rate and depth

7. Metabolic acidosis is a condition in which there is an increase in hydrogen ion concentration in ECF that is secondary to an increase in acids produced by the metabolizing of nutrients.
Possible causes of metabolic acidosis include all of the following EXCEPT

   A. gastric suctioning and emesis
   B. keto-acidosis
   C. high fat diet and excessive alcohol intake
   D. renal tubular acidosis

8. _____ is NOT an age-related change in the gastrointestinal tract.

   A. Decreased taste sensation
   B. Increased gastric secretion
   C. Loss of elasticity in the intestinal wall and slower motility
   D. Decreased blood flow to the intestines

9. Fluid and electrolyte balance in elderly people has been disturbed in many ways.
All of the following age-related changes in the urinary system affect fluid and- electrolyte balance EXCEPT

   A. decreased renal blood flow
   B. chronic residual urine predisposing to infection
   C. increased bladder capacity
   D. delayed excretion of water-soluble medications

10. Septic shock is the most common form of distributive shock, associated with a severe, overwhelming infection. Of the following, the one which is NOT among the gram negative organisms involved in the causation of septic shock is

    A. klebsiella-enterobacter-serratia
    B. escherichia coli
    C. rickettsiae
    D. pseudomonas aeruginosa

11. Almost half of all cases of septic shock develop in patients over 65 years of age. Elderly patients are at an increased risk for septic shock because

    A. elderly patients may not be able to clear their airways because of decreased mucociliary function
    B. poor nutrition and general debilitation can weaken the respiratory muscles
    C. limited activity and a sedentary lifestyle can lead to skin breakdown, which serves as a portal of entry for invading microorganisms
    D. all of the above

12. In some cases of cardiogenic shock, pharmacologic measures fail. The other method utilized to improve the pumping action of the heart is intra-aortic balloon counterpulsa-tion. All of the following are advantages of intra-aortic balloon counterpulsation EXCEPT

    A. increased myocardial oxygen supply as a result of improved coronary artery perfusion
    B. it is especially useful in aortic valve abnormalities
    C. decreased myocardial oxygen consumption
    D. relief of pulmonary congestion

13. Along with definitive therapy specific to each type of shock, which of the following supportive measures should be adopted to maintain adequate tissue perfusion?

    A. Establishment of adequate ventilation and oxygena-tion
    B. Restoration of optimum intravascular volume
    C. Maintenance of adequate cardiac output
    D. All of the above

14. Anaphylactic shock occurs as an allergic response to foreign antigens. Nursing care of a patient in anaphylactic shock would involve all of the following EXCEPT

    A. obtaining a careful, detailed allergic history
    B. rapid administration of drugs to avoid any additional allergic reactions
    C. exploring the patient's signs and symptoms
    D. carefully typing and matching the blood if a transfusion becomes necessary

15. Intra-arterial blood pressure can be directly measured using an in-dwelling catheter, usually inserted into the radial artery. Among the disadvantages of an intra-arterial catheter is

    A. damage to the arterial wall as a result of excessive flushing of the line or manipulation of the arterial catheter
    B. infection related to frequent manipulation of the arterial catheter
    C. ischemia distal to the insertion site
    D. all of the above

16. A pulmonary artery catheter is used for monitoring shock. All of the following are possible complications associated with the pulmonary catheter EXCEPT a(n)

A. disturbance in cardiac rhythm as a result of the presence and motion of the catheter
B. dilatation of the pulmonary artery with an increase in pulmonary blood flow
C. rupture of the pulmonary vessel due to overinflation of the balloon
D. increased susceptibility to infection

17. A patient in cardiogenic shock has decreased cardiac output as a result of the loss of the functional heart muscle.
Nursing intervention should include

   A. continuously monitoring the patient's arterial blood pressure and cardiac rhythm
   B. obtaining hemodynamic pressure measurement of right atria pressure, pulmonary artery pressure, cardiac output, and PWP
   C. maintaining the patient on modified bedrest or activity restriction to minimize the myocardial oxygen demand
   D. all of the above

18. A patient generally requests analgesics after the pain has begun.
Advantages of scheduled around-the-clock analgesics include all of the following EXCEPT

   A. decreased dosage since analgesics are most effective if given before the pain occurs or becomes severe
   B. decreased anticipatory pain
   C. patient being put in a dependent position of having to request pain medication after the pain has begun
   D. decreased anxiety about pain medication

19. Continuous subcutaneous opiod infusion is a useful alternative for a patient who prolonged the administration of parenteral opiods.
It is an advantage of continuous subcutaneous opiod infusion that

   A. there is no delay in drug administration
   B. it avoids repetitive injections and the need for IV access
   C. it avoids peak and trough drug levels
   D. all of the above

20. Proper nursing care of a patient with continuous subcutaneous opiod infusion would NOT include

   A. inspecting the site every shift for signs of irritation
   B. changing the site every other day
   C. monitoring for signs and symptoms of toxicity
   D. instructing the patient and the patient's family about the procedure and the pump

21. Spinal administration of opiods is usually reserved for patients with severe cancer pain who have tried adequate dosages of opiods by other routes without obtaining relief. Possible side effects of spinal administration of opiods include all of the following EXCEPT

   A. nausea and vomiting
   B. pruritis and sedation
   C. polyurea
   D. respiratory depression

22. Nursing care of patients with epidural opiod analgesia would NOT necessarily include

   A. close monitoring of the patient after catheter insertion, as respiratory depression may occur up to 24 hours after insertion
   B. a short-acting barbiturate made readily available as an opiod antagonist
   C. vital signs taken every 30 minutes
   D. checking for signs of redness and swelling at the insertion site, as meningitis may occur

23. Trans-cutaneous electrical nerve stimulation has been used as a non-invasive pain control measure for almost 20 years.
   The one of the following which contraindicates trans-cutaneous electrical nerve stimulation is

   A. chronic benign phantom limb pain
   B. confused or elderly patients with decreased sensory perception
   C. pregnancy in the first trimester
   D. patients with histories of cardiac dysrhythmias or myocardial infarctions

24. A stellate ganglion block is a type of nerve block requiring the injection of a local anesthetic agent into a sympathetic nerve group.
   All of the following are indications for stellate ganglion block EXCEPT

   A. pain in face, shoulder, head, and neck
   B. acute herpes zoster
   C. phantom lower limb pain
   D. postherpetic neuralgia

25. Regarding geriatric considerations in pain management, it is NOT true that

   A. elderly patients have a lower tolerance for cutaneous pain but an increased tolerance for deep pain
   B. depression can also masquerade as pain
   C. the elderly are at higher risk for drug-related toxicity than younger adults due to multi-drug interactions and decline in the function of organs such as the kidneys
   D. disorders such as musculoskeletal disorders, heart diseases, and cancer are more prevalent in the elderly and produce pain

26. Most pain clinics accept patients on a referral basis and may be either outpatient or inpatient clinics.
   All of the following are goals of most pain clinic teams EXCEPT to

   A. decrease the patient's degree of pain
   B. increase the patient's dependency on pain medications
   C. increase the patient's activity and ability to function
   D. improve the patient's sleep

27. Certain dietary fats may enhance the production of carcinogens by increasing the amount of bile acids and cholesterol metabolites in stool.
   Of the following malignancies, high fat intake is NOT associated with

   A. naso-pharyngeal carcinoma
   B. carcinoma of the breast
   C. colonic cancer
   D. carcinoma of the prostate

28. All of the following are tumors originating in the underlying epithelium EXCEPT the

    A. hydatiform mole   B. leiomyosarcoma
    C. adenocarcinoma   D. basal cell carcinoma

29. A 75-year-old black male is found to have a prostatic carcinoma. All of the following are common metastatic sites for carcinomas EXCEPT the

    A. bone   B. lungs   C. skin   D. liver

30. The use of tobacco products currently causes more than 30% of cancer deaths. Reduction of its use would have a significant impact.
Nurses play a key role in reducing tobacco use by

    A. educating the public regarding the hazards of tobacco
    B. assisting a patient with smoking-cessation activities
    C. promoting a smoke-free environment and smoking cessation programs within work environment
    D. all of the above

KEY (CORRECT ANSWERS)

1.	B	16.	B
2.	C	17.	D
3.	B	18.	C
4.	C	19.	D
5.	B	20.	B
6.	C	21.	C
7.	A	22.	B
8.	B	23.	A
9.	C	24.	C
10.	C	25.	A
11.	D	26.	B
12.	B	27.	A
13.	D	28.	B
14.	B	29.	C
15.	D	30.	D

TEST 2

DIRECTIONS: Each question or incomplete statement is followed by several suggested answers or completions. Select the one that BEST answers the question or completes the statement. *PRINT THE LETTER OF THE CORRECT ANSWER IN THE SPACE AT THE RIGHT.*

1. A 55-year-old post-menopausal woman is diagnosed as having an ovarian carcinoma. The tumor marker present specifically for ovarian carcinoma is   1.____

    A. carcino-embryonic antigen
    B. CA-125
    C. alpha-feto protein
    D. immunoglobulins

2. Education is the key to the successful screening and detection of a tumor. Nurses play an important role in cancer prevention and detection by providing education regarding   2.____

    A. techniques of self-examination of the breasts, skin, and testicles
    B. dietary modification, smoking cessation, and weight control
    C. the importance and proper frequency of screening tests
    D. all of the above

3. When a patient is receiving radiation therapy, the skin in the area being treated must be given special care. Nurses should tell the patient to do all of the following EXCEPT   3.____

    A. expose the treatment area to sun
    B. not use any creams, deodorants, or lotions on the area unless it has been provided by a concerned physician
    C. not wear constrictive clothing over the area
    D. not scratch dry and itchy skin but rather inform a physician so that a topical medication can be prescribed

4. Common gram negative bacteria that cause infection in elderly immunocompromised patients with cancer do NOT include   4.____

    A. pseudomonas
    B. cornybacteria and enterococci
    C. klebsiella pneumonia
    D. escherichia coli and proteus

5. A 62-year-old white male with an underlying malignancy develops disseminated intravascular coagulation.
All of the following are risk factors for DIC EXCEPT   5.____

    A. acute leukemia
    B. adeno-carcinoma of the prostate
    C. bone metastases
    D. sepsis and liver failure

6. Nursing care of the patient described in the above question should include   6.____

    A. administration of heparin and epsilon amino caproic acid
    B. blood product replacement and frequent monitoring of vital signs
    C. protection from further bleeding or trauma
    D. all of the above

7. The diagnosis of cancer has profound effects on patients and their families, especially in older patients who may have already lost several family members and friends to cancer. During the diagnostic and treatment phases, nurses should provide

   A. positive feedback and reinforcement regarding successful participation in self-care
   B. encouragement of activities that foster self-esteem, such as improvement of physical appearance, return to work and return to family roles and activities
   C. exploration and encouragement of useful coping strategies, including exercise and relaxation techniques
   D. all of the above

8. To reduce the suffering associated with the physical, emotional, or interactive aspect of a terminally ill patient, a nurse should perform all of the following activities EXCEPT

   A. physiologic care, such as activities of daily living
   B. spiritual aspects, such as facilitating participation in worship services and praying with the patient
   C. psychologic care, including touching and listening
   D. none of the above

9. Vitamin A is a fat-soluble vitamin which helps in the development and maintenance of epithelial tissues.
   A deficiency of Vitamin A is manifested in all of the following ways EXCEPT

   A. hemolytic anemia
   B. night blindness
   C. dry skin and poor skin healing
   D. respiratory infection

10. A 58-year-old female is on tube feeding.
    Possible complications of enteral tube feeding do NOT include

    A. pulmonary aspiration of formula
    B. pseudomembranous colitis
    C. hyperglycemia and electrolyte imbalance
    D. diarrhea

11. A nurse taking care of a patient with tube feeding should play a role in preventing and managing the above-mentioned complications through

    A. frequent assessment of the patient's status and response to tube feeding
    B. the monitoring of physical and laboratory data
    C. consultation with the physician and other health care team members to alert them to any potential problems
    D. all of the above

12. As the TPN catheter is an in-dwelling foreign body, it represents a major potential source of infection.
    In order to detect infection early and intervene appropriately, a nurse should do all of the following EXCEPT

    A. change the TPN catheter dressing, tubing, and solution under aseptic conditions
    B. inspect the solution for cloudiness, cracks, or leaks before hanging
    C. always draw blood or administer other fluids or medications via the TPN catheter
    D. change the TPN dressing if it becomes wet, soiled, or non-adherent

13. In preparing a patient and his family to deliver tube feeding safely at home, the nurse should advise them to report _____ to the health care team.

    A. diarrhea persisting more than 2-3 days
    B. difficulty breathing, rapid respirations, or frothy sputum
    C. a consistent average weight gain of more than half a pound per day over several days
    D. all of the above

14. An effective weight loss regimen requires major changes in deeply ingrained eating habits and lifestyle.
    The nurse planning weight reduction in an overweight patient must do all of the following EXCEPT

    A. establish with the patient long-term and immediate weight goals
    B. make permanent eating and lifestyle changes
    C. set a long-term goal of the loss of 75 lbs. of weight in one month
    D. achieve and maintain the target weight

15. In the patient education guidelines for weight control, all of the following statements regarding exercise are true EXCEPT:

    A. Use large muscle groups in sustained activity
    B. Utilize at least 300 calories per session
    C. Exercise at least 5 days a week
    D. Increase energy expenditure during daily activities

16. *Sensory deprivation* is a state in which the level of sensory input is insufficient to maintain the degree of cortical arousal necessary for homeostasis.
    Possible risk factors for sensory deprivation are

    A. spinal cord injuries and peripheral neuropathies
    B. aging and physical debilitation
    C. visual and hearing losses
    D. all of the above

17. *Sensory overload* is defined as a situation in which an individual is bombarded by multi-sensory stimuli at a greater than normal level of intensity.
    Desired outcomes for the nursing plan of care of sensory overload include all of the following EXCEPT that the patient will

    A. remain alert and oriented to the physical environment
    B. not verbalize decreased anxiety or irritability
    C. engage in meaningful conversation
    D. respond appropriately to environmental stimuli

18. *Insomnia* is the most common sleep disorder, occurring most frequently in women and the elderly.
Sleep deprivation leads to all of the following physiologic conditions EXCEPT

    A. increased respirations
    B. cardiac arrhythmias
    C. loss of equilibrium
    D. slow reflexes

19. Nurses institute all of the following measures to promote adequate sleep periods EXCEPT

    A. managing dietary and chemical substance intake
    B. using monitoring techniques that maximize the need to awaken the individual
    C. minimizing nighttime noise and treatment
    D. maintaining a cycle of light and darkness

20. The outcome criteria for nursing intervention in a patient with sleep pattern disturbance includes that the individual

    A. carries out measures to promote sleep
    B. has undisturbed periods for sleep
    C. reports feeling rested upon awakening
    D. all of the above

21. While educating a patient with sleep pattern disturbances, a nurse should state all of the following guidelines for developing good sleeping habits EXCEPT:

    A. Maintain the same daily schedule for waking, resting, activity, and sleeping 7 days a week
    B. Control the ambient temperature, noise, and light in your bedroom, if possible
    C. Do not eat a meal within 5 hours of bedtime
    D. Use your bed only for sleep-compatible activities

22. Direct expression of anger, whether verbal, nonverbal, or physical, may produce a feeling of helplessness or anxiety in a nurse.
Novaco observed the positive function of anger expression that

    A. anger can serve as a defense for feelings of anxiety
    B. anger gives an individual a sense of control over a situation and alleviates his sense of helplessness
    C. open expression of anger is characteristic of a healthy relationship
    D. all of the above

23. The care of dependent and manipulative patients can be frustrating for a nurse.
In order to give the best care to these patients, a nurse should NOT

    A. stay nonjudgmental, calm and objective
    B. make 1 or 2 long visits to the patient
    C. use a kind but very firm matter-of-fact attitude
    D. provide an outlet for anger, such as art, music, projects, or reading

24. *Self-concept* is the mental image or picture of the self. Loss of control and independence seems to be the greatest threat to the elderly and their self-concepts.
    To help avoid these problems, nurses should try to

    A. concentrate on preserving physical functions and give the patient choices whenever possible
    B. enhance the patient's self-esteem by promoting self-care and social relationships
    C. maintain the patient's independence by providing support services such as transportation, meals on wheels, and home health aids
    D. all of the above

25. Nursing intervention in the case of a patient with an altered self-concept involves all of the following patient-education guidelines EXCEPT

    A. encouraging staff, family, and others to provide an environment of acceptance and care
    B. strongly discouraging patients to express their fears, feelings, concerns, and anger
    C. providing emotional, informational, and technical support and reassurance
    D. involving patients in as much self-care as possible

26. The feelings and emotions associated with loss are clinically identified as *grief*.
    Of the following, the one which is NOT a physiologic manifestation of grief is

    A. weight gain and excessive sleep
    B. lack of strength and physical exhaustion
    C. loss of libido or hyperactive sex drive
    D. feeling of a lump in the throat

27. A dying person has certain rights and needs which, if respected, can make their final years, months, and days manageable.
    The dying person's bill of rights includes which of the following statements?

    A. I have the right to be treated as a living human being until I die.
    B. I have the right to express my emotions and feelings about my approaching death in my own way.
    C. I have the right to be free of pain.
    D. All of the above

28. The term *hospice* has come to mean a philosophy of care for the terminally ill.
    The purposes and goals of hospice nursing are reflected by which of the following functions?

    A. Re-orient the patient and his family to the reality that home is the primary place for care.
    B. Restore the patient's uniqueness and his place in life.
    C. Re-educate the patient and his family to enable the dying individual to live as meaningful a life as possible in the remaining time.
    D. All of the above

29. To maintain the health and abstinence from substance abuse of a discharging patient, the nurse should advise him to

    A. eat three meals a day, selecting food from every food group
    B. avoid alcohol, which is high in calories and suppresses the appetite
    C. avoid caffeine and high sugar snacks as craving substitutes
    D. all of the above

30. It has been estimated that more than 60% of the operations performed in the United States could be done satisfactorily on an outpatient basis.
    A DISADVANTAGE of outpatient surgery is

    A. decreased exposure to hospital infection
    B. more psychological stress than is associated with hospitalization
    C. the patient may return to work earlier
    D. economic savings and consumer satisfaction

KEY (CORRECT ANSWERS)

1.	B	16.	D
2.	D	17.	B
3.	A	18.	A
4.	B	19.	B
5.	C	20.	D
6.	D	21.	C
7.	D	22.	D
8.	D	23.	B
9.	A	24.	D
10.	B	25.	B
11.	D	26.	A
12.	C	27.	D
13.	D	28.	D
14.	C	29.	D
15.	C	30.	B

EXAMINATION SECTION
TEST 1

DIRECTIONS: Each question or incomplete statement is followed by several suggested answers or completions. Select the one that BEST answers the question or completes the statement. *PRINT THE LETTER OF THE CORRECT ANSWER IN THE SPACE AT THE RIGHT.*

1. Cold can be a problem for older patients when the temperature drops below _____ °F.
   A. 78   B. 75   C. 68   D. 60

2. The inability to use objects correctly is known as
   A. ataxia   B. apraxia   C. aphasia   D. aphonia

3. A disturbance of the swallowing mechanism which may be due to neoplasms, inflammatory lesions, or neurological disorders is
   A. ataxia   B. apraxia   C. aphasia   D. dysphagia

4. An impaired peristaltic activity with tertiary contractions as is seen in older patients is known as
   A. presbyopia   B. presbycardia
   C. presbycusis   D. presbyesophagus

5. A bone loss of _____% is needed to be seen on radiographs.
   A. 5   B. 10   C. 20   D. 50

6. Which of the following is a common fracture site in the elderly?
   A. Hip   B. Skull   C. Sternum   D. Knee

7. Paget's disease is seen more frequently in _____ and is rare below age _____.
   A. males; 40   B. males; 75
   C. females; 40   D. females; 75

8. In elderly people, the center of gravity moves from the _____ to the _____.
   A. hips; neck   B. hips; upper torso
   C. knees; hips   D. knees; upper torso

9. Hospice is best seen as a _____ response to death and dying.
   A. belief   B. bereavement
   C. organizational   D. role

10. About what percentage of the American population over the age of 85 is confined to long-term care facilities?
    A. 1%   B. 5%   C. 20%   D. 55%

11. Kuebler-Ross had indicated that even throughout all of her stages of dying, the patient/client would

    A. continue to bargain
    B. continue to deny his status
    C. maintain some hope
    D. remain angry

12. A disease that reflects death, and thus carries a certain stigma in American society, is

    A. cardiac disease
    B. cancer
    C. diabetes
    D. hypertension

13. The power of an individual to be involved in his or her own care to the greatest extent possible reflects the doctrine of

    A. autonomy   B. beneficence   C. justice   D. veracity

14. The caregivers in American society who have the greatest interaction with the dying elderly are

    A. physicians
    B. psychologists
    C. nurses
    D. social workers

15. The initial step that must be dealt with in educational programs to teach health professionals about death and dying is

    A. becoming aware of the family's feelings and reactions
    B. becoming aware of one's own feelings and reactions
    C. psychological views of death and dying
    D. sociological views of death and dying

16. Which of the following groups has been shown in studies to think less often about death, but have a greater death fear than others?

    A. Critically ill individuals
    B. Lay public
    C. Physicians
    D. Nurses

17. When the patient/client is going to die, but does not know it, while everyone else around him does (e.g., nurses, family members), this would be classified as

    A. closed awareness
    B. mutual pretense
    C. open awareness
    D. suspected awareness

18. When the patient/client is going to die, and everyone involved knows it, but this is not discussed, this is known as

    A. closed awareness
    B. mutual pretense
    C. open awareness
    D. suspected awareness

19. Which institution did Benoliel classify as a *custodial institution for the prolonged dying of individuals with low social value*?

    A. Adult day care
    B. Hospice
    C. Hospitals
    D. Nursing homes

20. Which role is associated with the expectations that an individual wishes to live, will take advantage of supportive measures, and will cooperate with the rules and routines of caregivers?
    _____ role.

    A. Dying	B. Medical	C. Nursing	D. Sick

21. The *caveat* or *loophole* in the patient/client's right to refuse treatment is that the patient must be

    A. competent	B. expert
    C. intelligent	D. rational

22. Which type of euthanasia involves committing an act that will result in an individual's death?

    A. Active	B. Involuntary
    C. Passive	D. Voluntary

23. Which type of euthanasia involves the omission of acts that might prolong an individual's life?

    A. Active	B. Involuntary
    C. Passive	D. Voluntary

24. The possibility that active euthanasia of the dying may lead to active euthanasia of those marginalized by society is the _____ argument.

    A. expansion
    B. linear
    C. see one, do one
    D. wedge or *slippery slope*

25. A widow who finds that she is unable following the death of her husband to enjoy the things she used to do is suffering from

    A. anhedonia	B. loneliness
    C. self-reproach	D. somatic symptomatology

KEY (CORRECT ANSWERS)

1. C
2. B
3. D
4. D
5. D

6. A
7. A
8. B
9. C
10. C

11. C
12. C
13. A
14. C
15. B

16. C
17. A
18. B
19. D
20. D

21. A
22. A
23. C
24. D
25. A

TEST 2

DIRECTIONS: Each question or incomplete statement is followed by several suggested answers or completions. Select the one that BEST answers the question or completes the statement. *PRINT THE LETTER OF THE CORRECT ANSWER IN THE SPACE AT THE RIGHT.*

1. The expectation of death has been called _____ grief.

    A. acute B. advanced C. anticipatory D. reality

2. Although the classification of grief as pathological may be controversial, which of the following would not fit into the category of pathological grief?

    A. Chronic B. Delayed C. Inhibited D. Intense

3. From a cross-cultural perspective, which one of the following is the most universal expression of grief among humans?

    A. Crying
    B. Sexual acting out
    C. Stoicism
    D. Wailing

4. Which of the following would be a poor strategy in comnunicating with an elderly individual with hearing difficulties?

    A. Modulating a higher pitched voice
    B. Modulating a deeper pitched voice
    C. Minimizing background noise
    D. Securing the individual's attention visually

5. Hypothermia may be induced in some elderly individuals with temperatures as high as _____ °F.

    A. 78 B. 68 C. 58 D. 48

6. Diverticulosis is

    A. an inflammation of diverticula
    B. the most common disease of the colon
    C. more likely to be found in men
    D. thought to be due to excessive dietary fiber

7. Which of the following is NOT true regarding pneumonia in the elderly?

    A. It is more likely to be found in men.
    B. It is commonly considered to be one of the COPDs (chronic obstructive pulmonary diseases).
    C. Lessened pharyngeal reflexes may lead to increased aspirations in the elderly.
    D. The incidence of pneumonia in long-term care facilities is about double that in the community.

8. The National High Blood Pressure Education Program defines combined systolic-diastolic hypertension as systolic greater than _____ mmHg and diastolic greater than _____ mmHg.

    A. 140; 80 B. 160; 90 C. 180; 90 D. 180; 100

9. Which of the following have been implicated in increasing the risk of acute renal failure in older people?
    I. Antibiotic therapy
    II. Dehydration
    III. Radiographic procedures using contrast media
   The CORRECT answer is:

   A. I, II   B. I, III   C. II, III   D. I, II, III

10. A metabolic disease characterized by the inability to break down purines is

    A. gout   B. osteoarthritis
    C. osteoporosis   D. rheumatoid arthritis

11. Degeneration with age, such as are seen in the female breast following menopause, or the thymus in both males and females, is also called

    A. atrophy   B. amastia
    C. integration D. involution

12. Increases in _____ and decreases in _____ have been implicated in the increased depression seen in older adults.

    A. monoamine oxidase and serotonin; norepinephrine
    B. norepinephrine; monoamine oxidase and serotonin
    C. monamine oxidase and serotonin; glucocorticoids
    D. norepinephrine; glucocorticoids

13. Which of the following ethnic groups is at greatest risk for stroke?

    A. African-Americans   B. Caucasians
    C. Hispanics   D. Japanese

14. Which of the following best describes delirium (as compared to dementia)?

    A. Does not resolve
    B. Abrupt onset
    C. Intact remote memory
    D. Labile/inappropriate mood/affect

15. Which of the following is NOT true regarding the skin/ integumentary system of the elderly?

    A. It is more easily broken, bruised, and damaged.
    B. Butterfly needles (instead of hypodermic needles) may lessen skin damage.
    C. The elderly have a decreased pain threshold.
    D. The speed of healing of their skin is longer.

16. The _____ theory is considered to be a genetic theory of aging.

    A. accumulation   B. autoimmune
    C. Hayflick's aging clock D. wear-and-tear

17. The theory that aging is due to the formation of unstable atons in the cell is known as the _____ theory.

    A. cross linkage
    B. deprivation
    C. free radical
    D. Hayflick

18. Which of the following is an accurate percentage reflecting *normal* shrinkage of the brain with age?

    A. 1-2%
    B. 7-10%
    C. 20-35%
    D. 40-50%

19. Most estimates indicate that the maximum life span for humans is in the range of _____ to _____ years.

    A. 60; 70
    B. 70; 80
    C. 80; 90
    D. 90; 100

20. The decrease of ability of the eye to focus on objects at varying distances is also known as decreased

    A. acclimation
    B. accommodation
    C. acuity
    D. adaptation

21. The change in sensitivity of the eye as a function of a change in illumination is known as

    A. acclimation
    B. accommodation
    C. acuity
    D. adaptation

22. Which of the following measures of rigidity has shown the LEAST increase with increasing age?

    A. Applicator-adaptation
    B. Motor-cognitive
    C. Personality-perceptual
    D. Psychomotor speed

23. The Age Discrimination in Employment Act (ADEA) protects workers between the ages of _____ and _____.

    A. 20; 70
    B. 40; 70
    C. 20; 80
    D. 40; 80

24. Which of the following are true?
    I. With age, there is a definite decrease in field intelligence.
    II. With age, there is no or little decrease in crystallized intelligence.
    III. There is no *training effect* that helps to maintain intelligence with age.
    The CORRECT answer is:

    A. I, II
    B. I, III
    C. II, III
    D. I, II, III

25. Higher education for older adults is often provided by the _____ approach.

    A. elderhostel
    B. hospice
    C. traditional educational
    D. *returning retiree*

KEY (CORRECT ANSWERS)

1. C
2. D
3. A
4. A
5. B

6. B
7. B
8. B
9. D
10. A

11. D
12. A
13. A
14. B
15. C

16. C
17. C
18. B
19. C
20. B

21. D
22. C
23. B
24. A
25. A

EXAMINATION SECTION
TEST 1

DIRECTIONS: Each question or incomplete statement is followed by several suggested answers or completions. Select the one that BEST answers the question or completes the statement. *PRINT THE LETTER OF THE CORRECT ANSWER IN THE SPACE AT THE RIGHT.*

1. Which of the following factors contributes MOST to the difficulty people experience in adjusting to retirement?

    A. Missing the work environment
    B. Death of a spouse
    C. Reduced income
    D. Declining health

2. Which of the following BEST illustrates *social* death?

    A. Talking about a dying person who is capable of hearing
    B. Bringing a dying person to a nursing home
    C. Helping a dying person to share his/her thoughts that are intimate
    D. Treating a dying person as a child

3. Which of the following groups tends to have the GREATEST fear of death?

    A. Sporadically religious people
    B. Atheists
    C. Strongly religious people
    D. Converts

4. Acceptance is the last stage in the dying process.
   Which one of the following sequences lists the first four stages in the CORRECT order?

    A. Anger, denial, depression, bargaining
    B. Anger, bargaining, denial, depression
    C. Denial, depression, anger, bargaining
    D. Denial, anger, bargaining, depression

5. Which one of the following is NOT a basic dimension of adult independence?

    A. Cultural   B. Economic
    C. Social   D. Physical

6. Approximately what percent of senior citizens are living in their own households?

    A. 80%   B. 90%   C. 60%   D. 70%

7. _____ is the process of getting over another person's death.

    A. Ageism   B. Disengagement
    C. Bereavement   D. Dependency

8. The degree of independence in old age is attributed to several key factors. Which one of the following is NOT considered to be a key factor?

    A. Finances
    B. Mobility
    C. Housing
    D. Religion

9. According to Barbara Anderson and Margaret Clark's book entitled CULTURE AND AGING, adaptation to aging is defined by various adaptive tasks.
   In their study of a San Francisco community, they found that the task to which more than half of the maladapted could NOT adjust was to

    A. substitute sources of need satisfaction
    B. accept the aging process
    C. revise criteria for self-evaluation
    D. integrate values and life goals

10. Approximately what percent of senior citizens have serious alcohol-related problems?

    A. 35%   B. 25%   C. 15%   D. 5%

11. Which of the following BEST describes the expression *dying trajectory*?
    The length of time between

    A. initial and terminal diagnoses
    B. a terminal diagnosis and death
    C. an initial diagnosis and recovery
    D. a healthy state and death

12. S.C.O.R.E. is an organization which helps owners of small businesses who are having management problems.
    What does the acronym S.C.O.R.E. stand for?

    A. Service Committee of Retired Educators
    B. Senior Council of Retired Engineers
    C. Senior Conference of Retired Employers
    D. Service Corps of Retired Executives

13. Approximately what percent of senior citizens have NEVER married?

    A. 3%   B. 10%   C. 17%   D. 25%

14. Which of the following meets all the conditions for a primary group formation?

    A. Hospital   B. Church   C. Family   D. School

15. The family life cycle, as defined by sociologists, contains several stages.
    Which of the following is NOT one of those stages?

    A. Marriage
    B. Bearing children
    C. Divorce
    D. Staying together until one spouse dies

16. Author Alan Kerckhoff was able to determine three norm value clusters associated with a family.
    Which of the following sequences describes these clusters in CORRECT order from least bonding to greatest bonding among family members?

    A. Modified, extended, nucleated
    B. Nucleated, modified, extended
    C. Modified, nucleated, extended
    D. Nucleated, extended, modified

16.____

17. Of all the senior citizens who get married each year, approximately what percent of these are first-time marriages?

    A. 5%   B. 10%   C. 15%   D. 20%

17.____

18. The two MOST important factors affecting marriage for older people are income and

    A. geographical location   B. gender ratio
    C. church affiliation   D. community involvement

18.____

19. Homogamy means the tendency for people of _____ backgrounds to _____.

    A. different; marry
    B. similar; divorce
    C. different; convert to the same religion
    D. similar; marry

19.____

20. Approximately how many older men are there for each 100 older women?

    A. 45   B. 60   C. 75   D. 90

20.____

21. Which of the following groups of older people has the HIGHEST mortality and suicide rates?

    A. Divorced   B. Married
    C. Never married   D. Widowed

21.____

22. Approximately what percent of senior citizens are great-grandparents?

    A. 30%   B. 40%   C. 50%   D. 60%

22.____

23. Approximately what percent of senior citizens have AT LEAST one living sibling?

    A. 30%   B. 45%   C. 65%   D. 80%

23.____

24. According to most sociologists, what is the accepted number of years which separates one generation from the next?

    A. 15   B. 20   C. 25   D. 30

24.____

25. The average number of children in a *completed* family is

    A. 1.6   B. 2.1   C. 2.6   D. 3.1

25.____

KEY (CORRECT ANSWERS)

1.	C	11.	B
2.	A	12.	D
3.	A	13.	B
4.	D	14.	C
5.	A	15.	C
6.	B	16.	B
7.	C	17.	A
8.	D	18.	B
9.	A	19.	D
10.	C	20.	C

21. A
22. B
23. D
24. B
25. C

TEST 2

DIRECTIONS: Each question or incomplete statement is followed by several suggested answers or completions. Select the one that BEST answers the question or completes the statement. *PRINT THE LETTER OF THE CORRECT ANSWER IN THE SPACE AT THE RIGHT.*

1. Approximately what percent of the world population are senior citizens (aged 65 or over)?

    A. 3%   B. 6%   C. 9%   D. 12%

2. Before the mid-1800's, the LARGEST compensating factor for the high annual death rate was the

    A. number of illnesses B. number of births
    C. population density   D. limit of available medicine

3. Approximately what percent of the United States population are senior citizens?

    A. 25%   B. 21%   C. 17%   D. 13%

4. When annual death rates fall from high unstable levels to low steady ones, this change is called an

    A. edacious transition B. effusive transfer
    C. epidemiologic transition D. endemic transfer

5. Which country has the SECOND largest elderly population?

    A. United States B. Great Britain
    C. India   D. China

6. Which of the following is a characteristic of a rectilinear age structure?

    A. Middle-age mortality increases
    B. Birth rate decreases
    C. Middle-age and old-age mortality are inversely related
    D. Early and middle-age mortality is low

7. The countries _____ and _____ are closer to population equilibrium than are other developed nations.

    A. Sweden; Switzerland B. France; Switzerland
    C. France; Germany   D. Germany; Sweden

8. Sociologists follow a general guideline that past the age of 30 the risk of death doubles every _____ years.

    A. 16   B. 12   C. 8   D. 4

9. In countries which are classified as *low-mortality*, cancer and _____ disease account for about 75% of all deaths for people aged 65 and older.

    A. lung   B. cardiovascular
    C. kidney D. intestinal

10. What is the concept of *pleiotropy*, as proposed by biologist George Williams in a paper on senescence?

    A. Individual genes are involved in multiple processes.
    B. Some genes create harmful physiological effects.
    C. Certain genes dominate other genes.
    D. Most genes are geared toward the fitness of the body.

10.___

11. The London biologist T.B.L. Kirkwood proposed the theory of *antagonistic pleiotropy* to explain senescence.
    According to his theory, senescence occurs directly as a result of which of the following?

    A. Evolution   B. Gene abnormality
    C. Fat tissue   D. Sexual reproduction

11.___

12. In studies on (non-human) primates, which method has been shown to slow down the aging process?

    A. Dietary restriction   B. Active sexual activity
    C. Climate control   D. Human contact

12.___

13. The French researcher Jean-Marie Robine and his colleagues have demonstrated that women in Western societies can expect to spend up to _____ % of their lives disabled.

    A. 35   B. 25   C. 15   D. 5

13.___

14. Which two social problems are recognized by gerontologists as the MOST difficult that an aging population will face in future years?

    A. Funding health care and social isolation
    B. Age-based entitlement programs and funding health care
    C. Social isolation and age-based entitlement programs
    D. Caring for relatives and fear of dying

14.___

15. The acronym O.B.S. describes the behavior deficiencies associated with senility.
    What do the initials O.B.S. mean?

    A. Oblique Behavior Syndrome
    B. Oblique Brain Syndrome
    C. Organic Brain Syndrome
    D. Organic Behavior Syndrome

15.___

16. One theory on aging is referred to as the *reservoir theory*. Which of the following accurately describes this theory?
    Each person('s)

    A. accumulates a given amount of energy in the first year of life
    B. body will eventually wear out, part by part
    C. ends life with a specific amount of vitality unused
    D. begins life with a limited amount of energy

16.___

17. Most research on aging involves cross-sectional studies. These studies involve comparing what elements?

    A. A particular group at different time periods
    B. Two or more age groups
    C. Two or more ethnic groups
    D. A particular segment of a population

    17.____

18. According to the United States Bureau of the Census, which one of the following minority groups has the HIGHEST percent in the over-65 category?

    A. Black B. Chinese
    C. American Indian D. Japanese

    18.____

19. In the year 1900, what percent of the United States population was aged 65 or older?

    A. 12% B. 9% C. 6% D. 3%

    19.____

20. What is recognized as the major source of income for MOST retired people?

    A. Medicare B. Annuities
    C. Social Security D. Insurance benefits

    20.____

21. Gerontologists agree that the MAJOR source of stress for elderly people is

    A. fatigue B. illness
    C. helplessness D. insecurity

    21.____

22. In the stages related to the process of dying, which of the following is considered the *middle* stage?

    A. Bargaining B. Depression
    C. Anger D. Denial

    22.____

23. The average life expectancy in this century has

    A. increased
    B. decreased
    C. stayed the same
    D. only increased in females

    23.____

24. As a general rule,

    A. men outlive women
    B. women outlive men
    C. both sexes have the same life expectancy
    D. there is no average life expectancy for either sex

    24.____

25. In the next 15 years, the population of senior citizens is expected to

    A. slowly decrease B. remain constant
    C. dramatically increase D. have greater longevity

    25.____

KEY (CORRECT ANSWERS)

1.	B	11.	D
2.	B	12.	A
3.	D	13.	B
4.	C	14.	B
5.	C	15.	C
6.	D	16.	D
7.	A	17.	B
8.	C	18.	B
9.	B	19.	D
10.	A	20.	C

21. C
22. A
23. A
24. B
25. C

EXAMINATION SECTION
TEST 1

DIRECTIONS: Each question or incomplete statement is followed by several suggested answers or completions. Select the one that BEST answers the question or completes the statement. *PRINT THE LETTER OF THE CORRECT ANSWER IN THE SPACE AT THE RIGHT.*

1. Which of the following is NOT universal among cultures? 1.____

   A. The aged are always a minority.
   B. Females always outnumber males.
   C. All older people are treated differently because they are old.
   D. Social mores mandate that older people must be segregated from the younger population.

2. Which of the following characterizes Erik Erikson's *crisis* central to old age? 2.____

   A. Intimacy versus isolation
   B. Ego identity versus identity confusion
   C. Generativity versus stagnation
   D. Integrity versus despair

3. Which theorist/researcher first examined the life review in relation to old age? 3.____

   A. Butler   B. Erikson   C. Freud   D. Levinson

4. The danger in stage theories of aging (as well as stage theories such as Kuebler-Ross's of death and dying) is to view them as _____ rather than _____. 4.____

   A. accurate; false
   B. false; accurate
   C. descriptive; prescriptive
   D. prescriptive; descriptive

5. Which theory holds that decreased involvement of elders in society is beneficial? 5.____

   A. Activity   B. Disengagement
   C. Learned helplessness   D. Life satisfaction

6. Which theory has been criticized for treating the elderly as if they were *already dead*? 6.____

   A. Activity   B. Disengagement
   C. Learned helplessness   D. Life satisfaction

7. Which theory can be critiqued for assuming that individuals perhaps have more control over their lives than they really do? 7.____

   A. Activity   B. Disengagement
   C. Learned helplessness   D. Life satisfaction

8. Which classification of death assumes that systems will no longer be able to regenerate themselves?

    A. Biological
    B. Brain
    C. Cerebral
    D. Clinical

9. Which one of the following dementias has been implicated as genetic in origin?

    A. Creutzfeld-Jakob disease
    B. Huntington's chorea
    C. Multi-infract dementia
    D. Normal pressure hydrocephalus

10. Korsakoff's syndrome is a dementia caused by

    A. infection
    B. intracranial mass
    C. toxicity
    D. vascular deficits

11. Depression can mimic dementia in a type of pseudodementia. Which of the following signs would characterize pseudo-dementia?
    I. Rapid onset/duration
    II. Vague complaints of cognitive loss
    III. Attention and concentration remain relatively intact

    The CORRECT answer is:

    A. I, II
    B. I, III
    C. II, III
    D. I, II, III

12. The development of a therapeutic community is used in _____ therapy.

    A. environmental
    B. milieu
    C. reality
    D. remotivation

13. The growing inability to suppress irrelevant stimuli with age is known as the _____ theory.

    A. central processing
    B. neural noise
    C. perceptual noise
    D. selective attention

14. Assuming that the healthy portion of an individual's personality can be activated via restructuring the environment is used in _____ therapy.

    A. environmental
    B. milieu
    C. reality
    D. remotivation

15. Which of the following is NOT true regarding tooth loss in the elderly? Tooth loss is

    A. correlated with lower incomes
    B. usually a result of lack of proper dental care
    C. inevitable in the elderly
    D. often due to pyorrhea

16. In the large intestine, cancer occurs most frequently in the

    A. left colon
    B. rectum
    C. right colon
    D. sigmoid colon

17. Which of the following is true regarding the presentation of osteomalacia (as opposed to osteoporosis)?

    A. Muscle weakness is rarely present.
    B. Axial bones are more commonly affected.
    C. No presence of skeletal pain.
    D. Abnormal values for serum calcium

18. In 1972, the act that generated a national program for one nutritionally planned hot meal a day, 5 days a week, for people age 60 and over was the

    A. Comprehensive Services Amendment to the Older Americans Act
    B. Commodities Distribution Program
    C. Food Stamp Act
    D. Home Health Services Act

19. Which of the following are correct regarding urinalysis in the elderly?
    I. Asymptomatic pyuria is uncommon and should be further evaluated.
    II. Asymptomatic bacteriuria is common.
    III. Hematuria is uncommon and should be further evaluated.
    The CORRECT answer is:

    A. I, II   B. I, III   C. II, III   D. I, II, III

20. Which one of the following laboratory tests should remain unchanged in the elderly (i.e., aging changes do not occur in its parameters)?

    A. Blood urea nitrogen
    B. Glucose tolerance
    C. Prostate specific antigen
    D. Sedimentation rate

21. Which of the following are true?
    I. Medicare Part A is hospital services insurance.
    II. Medicare Part B is medical services insurance.
    III. Fees are charged for both Parts A and B.
    The CORRECT answer is:

    A. I, II   B. I, III   C. II, III   D. I, II, III

22. Title XX of the Social Security Act covers

    A. day care
    B. hospital services
    C. legal services and counseling
    D. medical services

23. Meals on Wheels programs are generally funded through

    A. Title III   B. Title XX   C. Medicare   D. Medicaid

24. Which of the following programs is capped at an annual appropriation level, requiring matching funds in cash or in kind?

    A. Title III   B. Title XX   C. Medicare   D. Medicaid

25. Which of the following is NOT true?

    A. Total spending for nursing home care for those age 65 and above is about evenly divided between public and private expenditures.
    B. Acute care is more often paid by third-party payers than long-term care.
    C. The major public funding sources for long-term care are Title XX and the Older Americans Act.
    D. Medicare does no funding of long-term care.

KEY (CORRECT ANSWERS)

1. D
2. D
3. A
4. D
5. B

6. B
7. A
8. A
9. B
10. C

11. B
12. B
13. C
14. D
15. C

16. B
17. D
18. A
19. C
20. A

21. A
22. A
23. A
24. A
25. D

TEST 2

DIRECTIONS: Each question or incomplete statement is followed by several suggested answers or completions. Select the one that BEST answers the question or completes the statement. *PRINT THE LETTER OF THE CORRECT ANSWER IN THE SPACE AT THE RIGHT.*

1. Which of the following best describes *compression of morbidity*? 1.____
    A. The postponement of death into advanced old age
    B. The postponement of disability and illness into advanced old age
    C. A reduction in death rates
    D. A reduction in disability and illness

2. The MAJOR funding source for adult day care is 2.____
    A. Medicaid   B. Medicare
    C. Philanthropy   D. Title III

3. Which of the following is an INSTRUMENTAL activity of daily living (IADL)? 3.____
    A. Bathing   B. Feeding   C. Shopping   D. Toileting

4. Which of the following is a Social Security Administration classification for relatives of elderly individuals unable to manage their financial affairs due to physical or mental impairment? 4.____
    A. Guardianship   B. Legal guardianship
    C. Power of attorney   D. Payee status

5. Which of the following is true? 5.____
    A. Fingernails are more prone to thicken with age than toenails.
    B. Most nail changes due to aging are due to diminished vascular supply.
    C. Nutritional status has not been implicated in age-related changes of the nails.
    D. Aging nails become less brittle and hard.

6. The primary etiology for pathological changes in aging skin is exposure to 6.____
    A. allergens   B. climate
    C. industrial contaminants D. sunlight

7. Shingles is also known as herpes 7.____
    A. melanogaster   B. simplex
    C. varicellae   D. zoster

8. A condition of older age in which there is excessive resorption and deposition of bone is 8.____
    A. osteoarthritis   B. osteomalacia
    C. osteoporosis   D. Paget's disease

9. In rheumatoid arthritis, morning stiffness lasts _____ with pain most severe in the _____. 9.____
    A. 10 to 30 minutes; morning
    B. 1 hour or longer; morning

87

C. 10 to 30 minutes; evening
D. 1 hour or longer; evening

10. A man over the age of 62 would probably be considered anemic if his hemoglobin was less than _____ g/100.

    A. 13   B. 15   C. 17   D. 19

11. The theory that holds that abused children may abuse their parents in later life is the _____ theory.

    A. dependency
    B. psychopathology of the abuser
    C. social learning (transgenerational)
    D. stressed caregiver

12. In elder abuse, the abuser is most likely a

    A. child caregiver   B. nurse or nurse's aid
    C. spouse   D. stranger

13. Which of the following is sometimes (unjustly) overlooked in assessments of the elderly and may explain behaviors such as inattention to bathing and malnutrition despite adequate foodstuffs?

    A. Kinesthesia   B. Olfaction
    C. Sensory overload   D. Touch

14. Which of the following is true regarding weight loss and gain in the elderly?

    A. Normal weight men tend to gain weight after age 70.
    B. Normal weight women tend to lose weight after age 70.
    C. Overweight individuals of both sexes tend to lose weight with age.
    D. Subcutaneous fat distribution does not change with age.

15. Which of the following is true regarding body composition changes with age?

    A. The specific gravity of the body increases with age.
    B. Fat concentration decreases by about 16 percent from age 25 to 75.
    C. Water content increases by about 8 percent from age 25 to 75.
    D. The extracellular component of water does not increase with age.

16. Which type of substance abuse is MOST common among the elderly?

    A. Amphetamines
    B. Alcohol
    C. Marijuana
    D. Over-the-counter and prescribed medications

17. Which of the following chronic dementias would probably be diagnosed by computed tomography or cisternography?

    A. Depression
    B. Hepatic encephalopathy
    C. Hypothyroidism
    D. Normal pressure hydrocephalus

18. Which of the following is among the most common causes of vertigo in older adults?   18._____

    A. Acoustic neuroma   B. Labyrinthitis
    C. Meniere's disease   D. Peripheral neuropathy

19. Which of the following statements is true?   19._____

    A. Upper respiratory infections are more common in the elderly.
    B. Lower respiratory infections are more common in the elderly.
    C. The pneumonia related mortality for individuals above 70 is 5 percent.
    D. The pneumonia related mortality for individuals above 70 is 50 percent.

20. The most common cause of iron deficiency anemia in older adults is   20._____

    A. blood loss   B. bone marrow dysfunction
    C. hemolysis   D. vitamin B_{12} deficiency

21. Almost all pulmonary emboli originate in the   21._____

    A. deep venous system of the legs
    B. superficial venous system of the legs
    C. heart
    D. lungs

22. The *dry mouth* that is seen in many elderly individuals is also known as   22._____

    A. asalivosis   B. dehystomia
    C. keratosis   D. xerostomia

23. Alternating episodes of bradycardia, normal sinus rhythm, tachycardia, and periods of   23._____
    long sinus pause during which the atria and ventricles are not stimulated to contract
    characterize

    A. atrial fibrillation   B. digitalis toxicity
    C. heart block   D. sick sinus syndrome

24. Which of the following conditions may be overlooked as some of its symptoms may be   24._____
    attributed to normal aging?

    A. Diabetes   B. Hyperthyroidism
    C. Hypothyroidism   D. Renal dysfunction

25. Fasting and the administration of enemas prior to some diagnostic tests can cause which   25._____
    of the following in the elderly?

    I. Dehydration
    II. Pseudodement ia
    III. Orthostatic hypotension

    The CORRECT answer is:

    A. I, II   B. I, III   C. II, III   D. I, II, III

KEY (CORRECT ANSWERS)

1. B
2. A
3. C
4. D
5. B

6. D
7. D
8. D
9. B
10. A

11. C
12. C
13. B
14. C
15. D

16. D
17. D
18. D
19. B
20. A

21. A
22. D
23. D
24. C
25. D

NURSING HOMES

CONTENTS

PART ONE: ASSESSMENT OF NEED: IS NURSING HOME CARE THE BEST ALTERNATIVE? 1
    What Are Some of the Alternatives? 1
    Where To Begin 4

PART TWO: SOME QUESTIONS ABOUT NURSING HOMES 5
    What Is A Nursing Home? 5
    What Kinds of Nursing Homes Are There? 5
    Why Do People Live in Nursing Homes? 6
    How Does Medicare and Medicaid Pertain to Nursing Homes 6
    How are Nursing Homes Owned and Managed? 8
    How are Nursing Homes Regulated? 8
    What Do Nursing Homes Do For Patients? 9
    Who Provides Care? 13
    What Rights Do Patients Have? 14

PART THREE: CHOOSING A NURSING HOME 17
    Planning Ahead 17
    Consulting Others 18
    Finding Out What Kind of Home Is Needed 18
    Deciding on the Location 19
    Locating Nursing Homes 19
    Narrowing the Field 20
    Visiting Nursing Homes 21
    Meeting with Key Personnel 21
    Checking with State Nursing Home Ombudsman 23
    Touring the Home 23
    Making Follow-up Observations 26
    Checking Costs and Other Arrangements 27
    Making the Decision 29
    Making the Selection 29
    Following up 30
    What To Do When You Have A Complaint 30

PART FOUR: CHECKLIST 31
    General Physical Considerations 32
    Safety 33
    Medical, Dental, and other Services 34
    Pharmaceutical Services 34
    Nursing Services 35
    Food Services 35
    Rehabilitation Therapy 36
    Social Services and Patient Activities 36
    Patients' Rooms 37
    Other Areas of the Nursing Home 37
    Financial and Related Matters 38

NURSING HOMES

PART ONE

Assessment Of Need: Is Nursing Home Care The Best Alternative?

When a person can no longer live independently, a decision must be made about the best alternative arrangement for care. Such a decision often must be made during a time of crisis—frequently when the patient is ready to leave the hospital after a serious illness or operation.

Changed care needs may arise because of many reasons. A person has a stroke and can no longer remain at home alone. Frequent falls cause broken bones, and the individual needs a more protective setting. Increased forgetfulness or a heart condition poses a potentially serious threat to the well-being of the individual and necessitates increased health supervision.

When an individual needs 24-hour care and supervision, a nursing home is probably the best answer. However, when a less intensive and less restrictive form of care will suffice, a mix of services and/or programs popularly called "alternatives to institutional care" may be more appropriate.

The first step is to find out—with the help of various experts—what level of care is actually needed, and then to determine what combination of services is required to meet this need. This is done through an assessment of needs: by the doctor to determine the medical needs; by the nurse to determine health and nursing needs; by the social worker to determine social needs; and by other experts such as the therapists (speech, physical, occupational) to determine any special needs. On the basis of these findings, a care plan is developed. The next step is to match the recommendations for care with appropriate services and programs in the community.

WHAT ARE SOME OF THE ALTERNATIVES?

While communities throughout the nation have made much progress in developing many different kinds of alternatives, not all

NURSING HOMES

of these services and programs are available in each community. So it is important to find out about what resources are available in your own community.

Descriptions of some of the alternatives that you might consider are:

Home Health Care covers a broad range of services that are brought to a person in his or her own home. It includes such services as:

- part-time skilled nursing care
- part-time services of home health aide and homemakers (made necessary by a patient's poor health)
- occupational therapy
- physical therapy
- speech therapy
- nutrition counseling
- some medical supplies and equipment

Home Health Aide Services are provided under the supervision of a professional therapist (who also assesses the person's needs and plans for the service to be provided).

A homemaker-home health aide carries out such tasks as assistance with bathing and dressing, meal preparation, light cleaning and laundry.

Chore Services include yard maintenance, snow shoveling and heavy cleaning, either alone or in combination with homemaker-home health aide services.

Home-Delivered Meals provide nutritious meals delivered to a person in his or her own home, if for some reason the person is unable to prepare meals. One or two meals a day may be provided. Most programs provide five meals a week, a few also provide meals on weekends.

Congregate (Group) Dining is where a nutritious noon meal is served to older persons at such sites as senior centers or schools. Participation in these programs affords the opportunity for social interaction and for planned social activities which may be offered by some of these programs before or after the meal. Many programs provide transportation.

Adult Day Health Care means an organized day program of therapeutic, social and health activities. Services are provided to adults with functional impairments, either physical or mental, for

NURSING HOMES

the purpose of restoring or maintaining the greatest capacity for self-care. Provided on a short-term basis, adult day health care serves as a transition from a health facility or home health program to personal independence. Provided on a long-term basis, it serves as an alternative to institutionalization in a nursing home in two ways: 1) when 24-hour skilled nursing care is not medically necessary; or 2) when institutionalization is viewed as undesirable by the individual or by his or her family.

Some Adult Day Care programs are primarily social in nature. Many of these programs provide some health supervision, establish linkages with community health facilities, or provide transportation to needed health services.

Transportation and Escort Services are provided through volunteer driver programs or special mini-bus services for elderly or handicapped persons who do not have private transportation or who are unable to use public transportation. Physical assistance is also provided to persons needing help in shopping, going to medical appointments, or for other activities.

Telephone Reassurance programs provide a daily contact for persons who live alone and who are anxious about their safety or security or have chronic health problems. Usually, the client calls a central switchboard at an agreed-upon time during the day. If no one answers a call placed to the home, the neighbors or the police are alerted to check on the person.

Friendly Visiting insures friendly contact made to persons who are isolated or homebound and do not have regular contact with relatives or neighbors. These visits are usually provided on a regular basis by volunteers from church groups or social agencies.

Protective Services provide legal and financial services and/or conservatorship (a type of guardianship) to mentally confused persons, and to others who are unable to manage their own affairs or protect themselves from injury or exploitation.

Elderly Foster Care is where a family or individual(s) share their home with an older person who is unable to live alone, usually due to a medical problem. Some states have programs which pay the foster family for giving care to an older person.

Congregate Living represents a shared living arrangement for several persons who can not live totally independently, but are able to live in a group, relying on the strengths each person can contribute to such tasks as cleaning, cooking and shopping.

NURSING HOMES

Sometimes, through pooling of funds, the group can afford to purchase housekeeping and cooking services that they could not afford if living in separate quarters.

Special Housing Arrangements are available in many communities for older or handicapped people. Many of these programs are for low and moderate income persons; some programs offer a variety of social and health-supportive services to the residents.

Hospice is a service, usually by a facility or at home, that provides supportive care for terminally ill patients (usually cancer victims) and their families, using an individualized plan of care approved by the family physician, especially to control and relieve pain. As needed, other kinds of home care are integrated into this service that is available on a 7 day a week, 24-hour basis.

Information and Referral services are designed to help the individual find where to obtain any of the needed services.

WHERE TO BEGIN

First, it is important to know about the facilities, programs, and services available in your community. You can be helped in this task by discussing the problem with the social services office of the community public welfare agency, the social worker in the hospital (if that is where the patient is at the time), or a social worker in any philanthropic or church-related social agency in your community. If there is a Information and Referral Service available in your community, this group can be of enormous help in providing guidance. The State Welfare Office (listed in the Appendix) can help you find your local welfare agency. Or you can contact your Area Agency on Aging for guidance. (The State Office on Aging, listed in the Appendix, can tell you where it is and give you the telephone number.)

Whenever possible, the assessment and planning process should involve all who are concerned—the individuals, the family, the physician, the social worker, and the clergyman.

As was mentioned earlier, many different types of care are now available to give you many more choices when long-term care problems arise. For some persons, however, nursing home care is the only answer to meet their needs. In those cases, the challenge is to find the most suitable nursing home for the individual and the family.

NURSING HOMES

PART TWO

Answers To Some Questions About Nursing Homes

WHAT IS A NURSING HOME?

In this guide, we use the term to mean a patient care facility that primarily provides nursing, medical, and rehabilitation care, but also furnishes residential and personal services as well.

Residential and personal services. These are the most basic services, ones that you would expect of most facilities for elderly people.

Residential care means providing a pleasant, healthful place to live—a comfortable room, nutritious meals, clean laundry, the services of a barber and beautician, and the companionship of others.

Personal care involves helping patients with such everyday tasks as dressing, bathing, toileting, eating and walking. It also includes certain kinds of supervision, such as helping patients to get to scheduled activities and therapy sessions, and helping them to follow prescribed programs of special diets and exercises.

WHAT KINDS OF NURSING HOME ARE THERE?

All facilities that can properly be called "nursing homes" do not offer the same level of care. Some homes specialize in personal care, while others specialize in health or nursing care. Others take care of residents with all kinds of needs—from help with eating to posthospital medical care. This situation became more clearly defined with the passage of Medicare and Medicaid legislation in the 1960's. These government programs established two categories of nursing homes (or long-term care facilities) according to the services they give:

> A *skilled nursing facility* (SNF) is a nursing home that has been certified as meeting Federal standards within the meaning of the Social Security Act. It provides the level of

NURSING HOMES

care that comes closest to hospital care with 24-hour nursing services. Regular medical supervision and rehabilitation therapy are also provided. Generally, a skilled nursing facility cares for convalescent patients and those with long-term illnesses.

An *intermediate care facility* (ICF) is also certified and meets Federal standards and provides less extensive health related care and services. It has regular nursing service, but not around the clock. Most intermediate care facilities carry on rehabilitation programs, with an emphasis on personal care and social services. Mainly, these homes serve people who are not fully capable of living by themselves, yet are not necessarily ill enough to need 24-hour nursing care.

Many nursing homes are certified to participate in both the Federal Medicare and Medicaid programs, and qualify as both skilled nursing facilities and intermediate care facilities.

WHY DO PEOPLE LIVE IN NURSING HOMES?

Many patients in nursing homes are old. Some are feeble and unable to take care of themselves and live safely on their own. Other patients, regardless of age, suffer from chronic illnesses and need some medical attention, but do not require hospital care. Still other patients have been transferred to the nursing home from a hospital to convalesce after a serious illness, accident or operation.

In recent years, nursing homes have received an increasing number of patients under the age of 65. Some of them are mentally retarded or have other developmental disabilities. Many of these younger persons as well as others have come to nursing homes from State mental hospitals. There are also a large number who are disabled war veterans or have permanent disabilities as the result of auto accidents or other trauma.

Some nursing home residents have no families. In other cases, the families are not able to supply the kind of care the individual needs—there may be no one home during the day, or the care needed may be too specialized or too expensive to provide at home. In still other cases, families may decide that keeping the person at home would upset family life too much.

HOW DO MEDICARE AND MEDICAID PERTAIN TO NURSING HOMES?

Created in 1965, these government programs are designed to help meet the health care needs and to help pay the bills of peo-

NURSING HOMES

ple over age 65 and the poor. Both programs include coverage for nursing home care. (It should be noted, however, that Medicare does not pay for care in an intermediate care facility.)

Medicare is a Federal program of hospital and medical insurance that applies to people over the age of 65, and also covers persons of all ages who have been disabled for at least two years or who have certain chronic renal disorders. It pays some of the cost of care in a skilled nursing facility. It covers a "spell of illness" of up to 100 days of care, but only after a stay of at least three days in a hospital. If care is needed beyond 100 days, the cost of care may be paid by Medicaid if the patient is eligible for such coverage. It is important to know that Medicare will not pay for care in a skilled nursing home unless the patient needs skilled nursing care or skilled rehabilitation services on a daily basis. Medicare cannot pay for care in an intermediate care facility, or for care in a skilled nursing home if the care needed is mainly custodial.

Care is considered custodial when it is primarily for the purpose of meeting personal needs and could be provided by persons without professional skills or training: Helping with such everyday tasks as walking, getting in and out of bed, bathing, dressing, eating, and taking medicine are considered custodial care.

Medicaid helps provide medical services to people with little or no income. The program is operated by the individual States (except for Arizona), although the Federal government provides up to 75 percent of the funds. Medicaid pays for care in both skilled nursing facilities and intermediate care facilities in all States (except Arizona); care in ICFs for the mentally retarded, is provided in most States. Since January 1, 1973, people who are medically needy share the cost of service they receive under Medicaid by paying a nominal enrollment fee or premium, based on the amount of the individual's income.

Medicare provisions change often, and Medicaid programs vary from State to State. For up-to-date information in your State, contact the local Social Security Office (for Medicare) or your State of local welfare office (for Medicaid). (Note: The telephone number for your local Social Security Office can be found in your telephone directory under U.S. Government. Addresses of the State welfare offices are listed in the Appendix.)

NURSING HOMES

HOW ARE NURSING HOMES OWNED AND MANAGED?

Some nursing homes are nonprofit institutions. They are sponsored by religious, charitable, fraternal and other groups or run by government agencies at the Federal, State or local levels. But most homes are private businesses, operated for profit. They may be owned by individuals or corporations. Sometimes they are part of a chain of nursing homes.

Final responsibility for the operation of a nursing home lies with its *governing body*. The governing body may be called the "board of directors" or "trustees," or they may be the owners of a proprietary facility. However they are constituted, they are the legal entity responsible for the home. The governing body meets periodically to set policies and to adopt and enforce rules and regulations for the health care and safety of patients.

The person in charge of the day to day management of a nursing home is called the *administrator,* and is appointed by the governing body. State licensing of the nursing home administrator is required.

HOW ARE NURSING HOMES REGULATED?

Nursing homes are required to meet standards set by State or local laws and regulations, and have a State license or letter of approval for a licensing agency to operate. *Participation by the nursing home in the Medicare and/or Medicaid programs is strictly on a voluntary basis.* Some nursing homes may choose to participate in only one program, and so are certified for that kind of program (Medicare or Medicaid); other nursing homes are certified for both Medicare and Medicaid. Payment for care in a nursing home by Medicare and Medicaid programs can be made only for care provided in certified facilities.

Nursing homes that are certified to take part in Medicare and Medicaid are required to meet standards set by Federal regulations. These standards are developed by the Bureau of Health Standards and Quality of the Health Care Financing Administration (HCFA), U.S. Department of Health and Human Services (DHHS).

HCFA is the agency responsible for continuing the Department's initiatives started in 1974 to improve the quality of care in long-term care facilities. As a part of this goal, a guide to patient care management has been developed which uses an integrated approach to patient care, and includes formal assessment of each patient's needs, a plan of care to meet those needs, and periodic evaluation of the outcomes of care.

NURSING HOMES

State agency or public health department surveyors evaluate homes periodically to make sure they meet health, safety, staffing and environmental standards, and that they are providing care that is consistent with the patient care management requirements.

WHAT DO NURSING HOMES DO FOR RESIDENTS

There is nothing about a nursing home that is more important than resident care. A home may be clean and well-equipped, but this means very little unless it also has a well-rounded program of good quality services for residents.

The goal of resident care in a nursing home is to provide care and treatment designed to restore and/or maintain the resident's highest level of physical and mental health.

Often nursing homes make arrangements with outside people to furnish certain services, such as rehabilitation therapy and consultation for dietary, social, activities and pharmaceutical needs.

The following pages describe some important aspects of care. (Additional points are covered in the checklist in Part Four.) Some of these points reflect Federal regulations for facilities participating in the Medicare and Medicaid programs. Others are simply good nursing home practices.

Food services. Residents should have meals that are nourishing, well-balanced, and appetizing. These meals should meet the daily nutritional needs of individual patients and should be properly scheduled. Residents should be offered nutritious snacks between meals and at bedtime. Some residents requrie special diets prescribed by their physicians. The facility should be able to provide such prescribed diets. Most often, food preparation takes place in the nursing home; in some cases, however, the nursing home makes arrangements with an outside company to provide food services. When you visit a nursing home, you will probably have a chance to meet the *food service supervisor* who is the person in charge of menu planning and food preparation. The kitchen staff should be large enough to prepare meals promptly and efficiently and under safe sanitary conditions. Hot foods should be served hot and cold foods cold.

Nursing services. In many ways, nursing care is what nursing homes are all about. Nursing personnel keep residents clean and comfortable, administer drugs, apply dressings and take steps to prevent pressure sores. They provide treatment to patients suffering from such problems as strokes, heart disease, and orthopedic illnesses who have been transferred from hospitals.

10
NURSING HOMES

When you visit a nursing home, you will see several kinds of people on the nursing staff:

> A *registered nurse* (RN) is a licensed nurse, usually having completed basic preparation in a diploma, associate degree, or baccalaureate degree program in an accredited school of nursing that requires two to four years of study. RNs supervise nursing services, carry out various administrative duties, and, as required to meet patient's needs, they are able to give highly skilled nursing care.
>
> A *nurse practitioner* is an RN with additional knowledge and skill gained through an organized nurse practitioner program of study and supervised practitioner experience. It is significant that after successfully completing graduate programs of study, an increasing number of professional nurses are awarded masters and doctoral degrees, and are thus prepared to assume broad nurse leadership and nursing care responsibilities.
>
> A *licensed practical nurse* (LPN) usually has had at least one year of specialized training. Generally, LPNs do the less complex nursing jobs, with emphasis on bedside care. In California and Texas, an LPN is called a *licensed vocational nurse* (LVN).
>
> *Nurses' aides* and *orderlies* work under the supervision of RNs and LPNs. They help residents get out of bed and get dressed in the morning, bathe them, make their beds, clean their rooms, bring their meals and feed them, and carry out similar kinds of personal care and housekeeping duties. Training of aides and orderlies is usually given by the nursing home.

Federal Regulations have very specific requirements for the nursing staff in nursing homes. These are covered in the checklist (Part Four.)

Physician services. Every resident in a nursing home must be under the care of a physician. A key role is played by the attending physician. He or she is responsible for the medical care of the individual patient—making the examination and diagnosis and prescribing the needed treatment, diet, drugs, and rehabilitation program. For the most part, the attending physician is the resident's own personal physician. In some cases, however, attending physicians are provided by the nursing home.

Federal regulations require that a skilled nursing facility must have a physician on its staff at least part-time to serve as medical

NURSING HOMES

director. The major functions of the medical director are: 1) coordinate all medical care for residents, 2) keep the quality of care under constant close watch, and 3) check on the health of the home's employees.

Federal regulations also set guidelines for visits by physicians. A resident must be given a physical examination just before or at the time he or she is admitted to the nursing home. Periodic follow-up visits should be made by the attending physician for continuous health management. In addition, good nursing homes bring in specialists to make regular checkups of residents' teeth, eyes, and feet. This is particularly important in care of the elderly.

Pharmaceutical services. Pharmaceutical services must be under the general supervision of a qualified pharmacist. A pharmacist reviews each resident's drug regimen regularly, and works with the physician and other facility staff to assure that each resident receives the right drug at the right time in the prescribed manner. Drugs are given to residents by qualified personnel, e.g., registered nurses, licensed practical nurses, or trained medication aides (under the supervision of a nurse).

Rehabilitation therapy typifies modern thinking about nursing home care. The principal aim is to help residents regain capabilities they have lost, allowing them to get along on their own as much as possible. Experience has shown that even the very elderly are often capable of great improvements.

Under Federal regulations, a nursing home may accept residents who are in need of specialized rehabilitation services only if it can provide or arrange for these special services.

Most nursing homes offer three types of rehabilitation therapy: *physical therapy, occupational therapy* and *speech/language pathology therapy.*

Physical Therapy. As a result of illness or injury, some people need help to regain lost abilities in body functioning. Physical therapists and their aides—using exercises, massages, and special training equipment—help residents to improve their abilities to sit, turn, stand, and walk or to carry on such everyday activities as eating, dressing and bathing. They also teach residents to use wheelchairs, braces, and artificial limbs.

When you visit a nursing home, you will probably see a special physical therapy room equipped with exercise equipment, whirlpool baths, and the like.

NURSING HOMES

Occupational Therapy. Occupational therapists work to develop occupational and recreational skills by involving residents in a variety of craft activities. These activities stimulate their interest and provide patients with a sense of satisfaction by accomplishing projects and by giving them practice in making precise movements of the hands and arms.

In large nursing homes, occupational therapy is usually carried on in a special room supplied with craft materials and equipment. In smaller homes, the dining room may double as an occupational therapy room.

Speech/Language pathology therapy. A speech/language pathologist helps residents overcome speech and language difficulties such as those due to stroke, hearing loss, or neuromuscular disorders. Speech/language therapy may be carried on in residents' rooms or in other areas of the home.

Social Services. Residents in nursing homes may have emotional concerns or problems and social adjustment difficulties. Sometimes these stem from entering the home itself: residents are separated from familiar people and places, their customary living patterns are disrupted, they are fearful of change and they become depressed. Sometimes the difficulties are connected with growing old, and feeling unwanted.

In recent years, we have come to realize more and more that nursing homes must deal with the whole person—not just with medical and physical needs, but with emotional and social ones as well. Nursing homes may not be required to offer social services themselves, but they are required to determine the social and emotional needs of the resident. If they do not provide these services to meet these needs, they must be able to refer residents and their families to outside agencies for assistance. If a home does provide social services, the person in charge is called the *director of social services*.

A good social service director tries to prepare people before they enter the home and help them adjust once they arrive. He or she counsels residents and their families, referring them to outside agencies for financial or legal help when necessary. When the time comes for residents to leave the nursing home, the director helps them and their families plan for the transition.

Reality Orientation: "Reality orientation" is a program which helps patients stay in contact with the real world by keeping them aware of the day and time of year, weather, holidays, activities in the home, and major news events.

NURSING HOMES

Patient activities. A suitable program of recreational activities in a nursing home is an important part of total care. Interesting and varied activities, supervised by a qualified activities coordinator, can do much to relieve the monotony of life and keep residents mentally alert, actively involved, and socially in contact.

Activities programs vary widely from one nursing home to another. Some homes have very limited programs. Others, particularly those with many active patients, have large and elaborate programs.

A well-rounded program may include individual activities (such as arts and crafts, reading, and letter writing), group activities (care games, billiards, exercise classes, drama and choral groups), noisy activities (rhythm bands, sing-alongs), highly social activities (dances, parties, birthday and holiday celebrations), outdoor activities (gardening classes, nature walks), and opportunities to get away from the home for a time (such as trips to parks, theaters, concerts, and museums).

Some nursing homes have book and record collections, movies, and discussion groups. Sometimes people from the community, such as librarians and theatrical groups, bring their services to the home. Some homes have a Resident Council which helps plan and carry on the activities program. A rich activities program is one of the hallmarks of a good nursing home, and you should inquire about it in any home you visit.

Volunteer program. A well-organized volunteer program can be a tremendous asset to a nursing home. Working and visiting with residents, community volunteers can help stretch a limited staff, increase the number of activities, and provide much needed contact with the outside world.

Religious observances. Many older people like to attend religious services and talk with clergymen. Nursing homes should provide opportunities to do so, whether in the home or at a nearby place of worship. Some homes have a chaplain and provide a chapel that is open for private meditation.

WHO PROVIDES CARE?

In a nursing home, each member of the staff plays a vital role in assuring that the resident receives a certain quality of care and services. The staff consists of administrative, professional, and non-professional personnel. The administrative staff is responsible for assuring that the facility operates effectively. Qualified health professionals, such as nurses, physicians, and dietitians,

NURSING HOMES

are responsible for assessing the needs of each resident and providing the necessary care. Professional staff are available to meet the medical, social, and emotional needs of each resident. The nonprofessional staff includes the aides and orderlies. These employees deliver many of the daily services directly to the residents in nursing homes.

Physicians, nurses, and other health personnel need to be attracted to providing long-term care in nursing homes. Today, education programs for health professionals frequently include both theory and practice in geriatrics and/or gerontology. These individuals will enter practice as better prepared and interested personnel.

WHAT RIGHTS DO PATIENTS HAVE?

Under Federal regulations, nursing homes must have written policies covering the rights of residents. They are required to make these policies available to residents and to the public. A kind of "bill of rights," the policies ensure that each resident admitted to the facility:

1. is fully informed, as evidenced by the resident's written acknowledgment of these rights and of all rules and regulations governing the exercise of these rights;

2. is fully informed, of services available in the facility and of related charges including any charges for services not covered under Medicare or Medicaid, or not covered by the facility's basic daily rate;

3. is fully informed, of his medical condition unless the physician notes in the medical record that it is not in the patient's interest to be told, and is afforded the opportunity to participate in the planning of his medical treatment and to refuse to participate in experimental research;

4. it transferred or discharged only for medical reasons, or for his welfare or that of other residents, and is given reasonable advance notice to ensure orderly transfer or discharge;

5. is encouraged and assisted, throughout his period of stay, to exercise his rights as a resident and as a free citizen. To this end he may voice grievances and recommend changes in policies and services to facility staff and/or to outside representatives of his choice without fear of coercion, discrimination, or reprisal;

NURSING HOMES

6. may manage his personal financial affairs, or is given at least a quarterly accounting of financial transactions made on his behalf if the facility accepts the responsibility to safeguard his funds for him;

7. is free from mental and physical abuse, and free from chemical and physical restraints except as authorized in writing by a physician for a specified and limited period of time, or when necessary to protect the patient from injury to himself or to others;

8. is assured confidential treatment of his personal and medical records, and may approve or refuse their release to any individual outside the facility;

9. is treated with consideration, respect, and full recognition of his dignity and individuality, including privacy in treatment and in care for his personal needs;

10. is not required to perform services for the facility that are not included for therapeutic purposes in this plan of care;

11. may associate and communicate privately with persons of his choice, and send and receive his personal mail unopened;

12. may meet with, and participate in activities of social, religious, and community groups at his discretion;

13. may retain and use his personal clothing and possessions as space permits, unless to do so would infringe upon rights of other patients, or constitute a hazard to safety;

14. is assured privacy for visits by his/her spouse; if both are inpatients in the facility, they are permitted to share a room.

NURSING HOMES

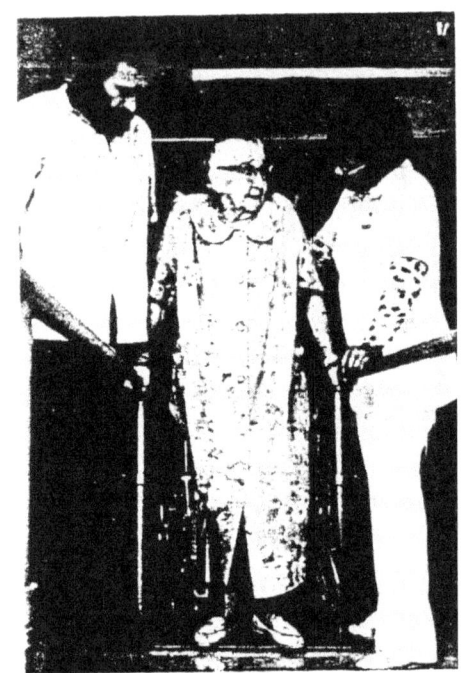
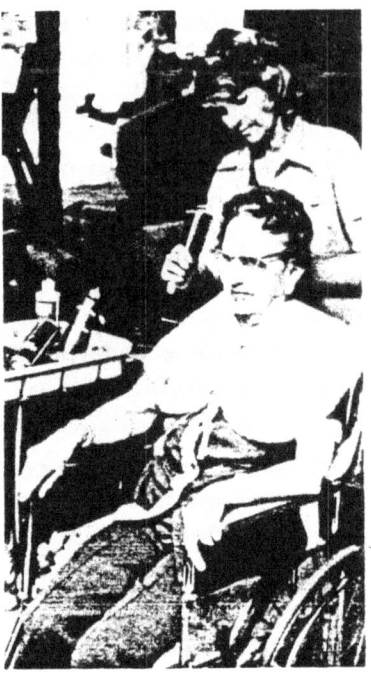
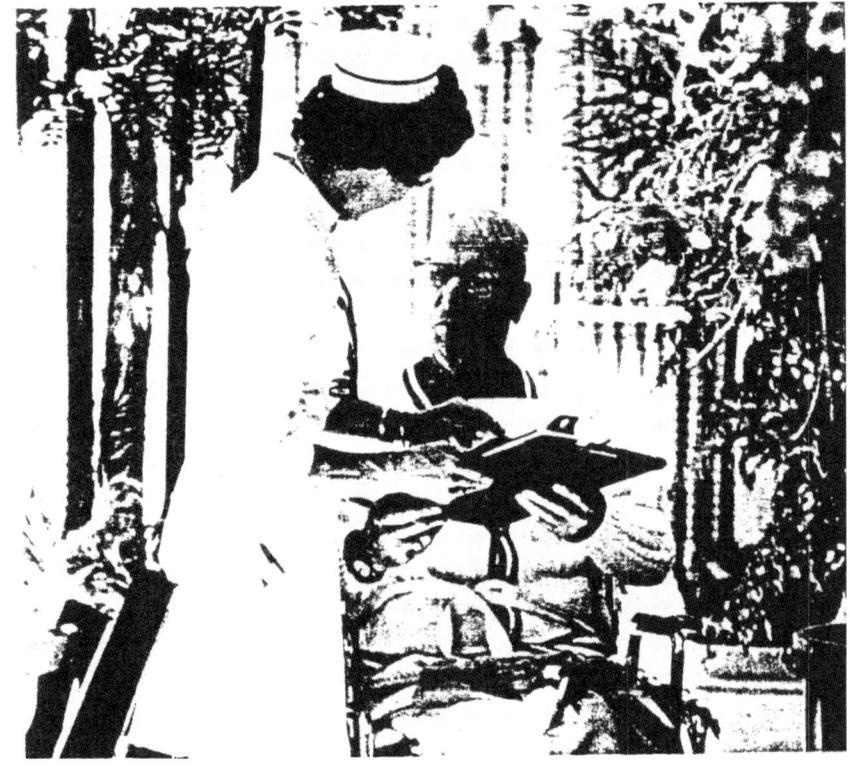

NURSING HOMES

PART THREE

Choosing A Nursing Home

PLANNING AHEAD. If you think you will need a nursing home at some time in the foreseeable future—for yourself or for an aging relative—it will pay to plan ahead. Many of the good nursing homes have long waiting lists, and chances of getting placement in the home of your choice may be greatly enhanced if placement is made on the waiting list prior to the actual time of need. Also this will give the prospective patient time to get mentally adjusted to the idea of the change.

Unfortunately, the choice of a nursing home is often made in a crisis atmosphere, when time is short and minds are troubled. But selecting a home is an important decision—one that deserves foresight and careful, clear-headed consideration.

Here are some things you can do in advance:

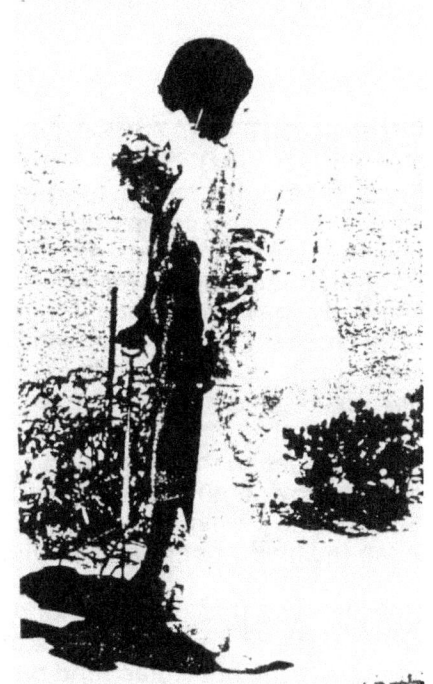

• Make a point of learning about nursing homes. In addition to reading this booklet, watch for articles in newspapers and magazines and for television programs that deal with nursing homes. Also, pick up brochures on the subject from social service agencies or your local health department.

• Find out what nursing homes are located in your community, and learn what you can about them. If you have friends or relatives who are familiar with the homes, ask for their opinions of them. If you know people who live in nursing homes, pay them a visit and gather some firsthand impressions.

NURSING HOMES

• Discuss the matter with the prospective patient, and find out his or her preferences.

• Think about ways of financing nursing home care. Find out whether the elderly person is likely to be eligible for Medicare or Medicaid or whether he or she has personal health insurance or a pension plan that covers nursing home costs. If not, begin planning other means of financing.

CONSULTING OTHERS. When the times comes to find a nursing home, other people can help. Consulting with the elderly person's physician is essential. Other physicians, social workers, clergymen, and friends or relatives who have placed someone in a nursing home can all offer valuable advice.

The person who will be entering the home should not be overlooked. If he or she is mentally alert, the person deserves to have his or her wishes considered and should be involved in the process of selecting the home every step of the way.

FINDING OUT WHAT KIND OF HOME IS NEEDED. The crucial question is: What kind of care does the elderly person need? Some may only require a safe and comfortable place to live, among pleasant companions. Some may want a home that places special emphasis on ethnic factors, such as special food or foreign languages; for some, there may be a preference for similarity in religious background. Others may need some help with grooming and occasional medical treatment. Still others may need constant medical attention, therapy, and other hospital-related care.

As discussed in the preceding section, different kinds of nursing homes provide different levels of care. The key is to match the home to the patient—to ensure the patient is in a home that provides the kind of care and services needed.

How can you find out what kind of care the person needs? The best source of guidance is his or her personal physician. When you talk to the physician, find out precisely whether an intermediate care facility or a skilled nursing facility can provide the level of care needed. Also ask about any special services or treatments that should be provided by the facility for the patient. (See p. 9).

NURSING HOMES

DECIDING ON THE LOCATION. In addition to finding out what *kind* of nursing home is needed, you should decide on a general location. In thinking about location, keep in mind that the most important goal is to provide the elderly person with the kind of care that is needed. Here are some points to consider:

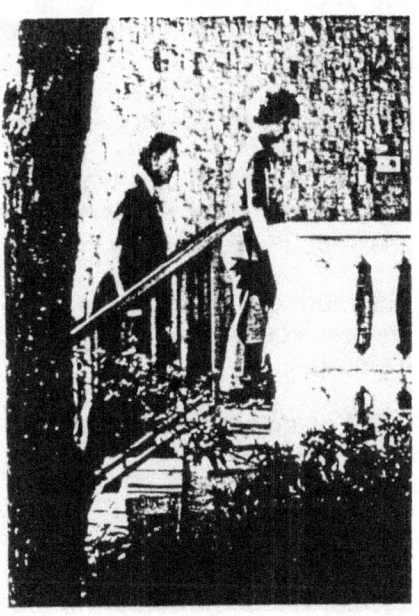

• The location should be agreeable to the elderly person. For example, some people may prefer the restfulness of country surroundings, while others may prefer the stimulation of city life and being near community services such as those available from churches or community centers.

• The home should be convenient for the person's family and friends. Having to make a long trip may discourage people who would otherwise visit often.
• The home should be reasonably close to a hospital offering emergency service. In the event of an emergency, reaching a hospital quickly may be crucial.

• If the available homes in the local area cannot meet the patient's needs, you probably should go further away to get it.

LOCATING NURSING HOMES. The next step is to find out which nursing homes are available in the area you have in mind. Go over the list with your physician to ascertain which nursing homes he would recommend.

Some communities now have citizen groups which visit nursing homes, compile directories of homes, make digests of survey reports, and in general, try to protect the consumer's interests. If there is such a group near you, it should be consulted.

Many agencies and organizations keep lists of homes in order to make referrals to the public. (Usually, however, they do not make specific recommendations.) These are some places you might contact:

- Local or State health department
- Hospital, Social Services Department

NURSING HOMES

- Provider associations, i.e., State Health Care Nursing Home Associations, Association of Homes for Aging, etc.
- Local Office of the Social Security Administration
- Local Welfare Department
- Church groups
- Yellow pages of your telephone directory

In addition, you can often talk to individuals who are acquainted with the nursing homes in a given area—people like physicians, clergymen, relatives, and friends.

Make a list of the homes mentioned to you. Do not worry if the list is long; the more choices you have, the better your chances are of making a good selection.

NARROWING THE FIELD. You do not need to visit all the nursing homes on your list. Some can be eliminated simply by making telephone calls to the homes.

Here are some things to ask about:

Does the home provide the kind of care the elderly person needs? Is the home of the kind specified by the physician—a skilled nursing facility, intermediate care facility, or whatever? Does the home supply the special services or programs the physician considers necessary?

Is the home approved for participation in the Medicare or Medicaid programs? If you will depend on financing through one of these programs, then obviously this is an important question. But even if you plan to pay your own bills, the fact that a home meets Federal as well as State standards should be a point in its favor.

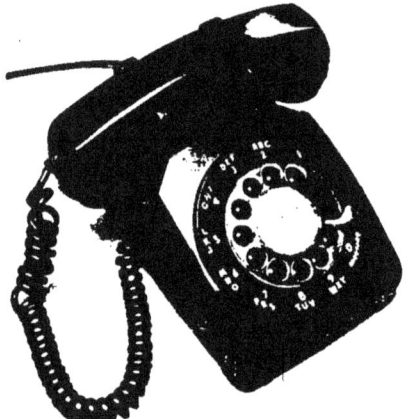

Does the home have an opening? If not, what is the likely waiting period? Many homes have waiting lists. Some put people on the list according to the date they apply. Others consider the elderly person's condition and the family's need to place the person in a home, and assign a position on the list accordingly.

What are the home's admission qualifications? Nursing homes vary widely in this respect. Some require that pa-

NURSING HOMES

tients be able to care for themselves to a certain extent. Some admit only patients who have been residents of the State. Some require proof or assurance in writing that you will be able to pay the bills. Some will not accept patients with serious mental disorders. Be wary of any nursing home representatives who insists that the patient sign over his personal and real property in exchange for care.

Getting recommendations. In addition to telephoning the nursing homes, try to find as many people as you can who are familiar with the homes on your list. Ask them which homes they do and do not recommend.

VISITING NURSING HOMES. By telephoning homes and getting people's opinions, you should be able to narrow the list. Now plan to visit each of them.

It is important to go to the homes in person *before* you make your choice. Only by seeing them firsthand can you get a true impression of the places and the people who work there. And only in this way will you be able to rest assured that you have made the best possible choice.

Because a nursing home is a complex operation, there are many things to find out when you visit. The following pages provide a general guide, with the emphasis on things to *do*. The checklist in the back of this booklet gives more specific points to look for and ask about. Take the booklet along and refer to the checklist during your visits.

Preparing for visits. For the first visit to a home, it is a good idea to make an appointment in advance. State that you would like to meet with the administrator—also, if possible, with the director of nursing services and the director of social services. Mention that you would like to watch a meal being prepared and served, and to see as many different therapy sessions and patient activities as possible.

Usually, a good time to visit is late morning or midday. By then the early morning cleanup is over and you will be in time for the noon meal.

A short time before your visit, review this booklet to refresh yourself on important points.

MEETING WITH KEY PERSONNEL. When you arrive at a home, spend some time with the administrator, the director of nursing services, and the director of social services. Talk with them long

NURSING HOMES

enough to get a feeling for the kind of people they are and their attitudes toward their work. Do not worry about imposing on their time, meeting with you and others like you is part of their job.

Encourage the people in the meeting to tell you about the history and philosophy of the home. Find out who owns the home and whether it is run on a profit or non-profit basis. (Under Federal regulations, the names of a home's owners and board members must be made available to the public.)

Verifying vital points. This is the time to check the state licenses or letter of approval from the licensing agency for the facility and for the administrator. Ask to see them, and look for dates to make sure the licenses are still in effect.

This is also the time to confirm that the home is certified for participation in the Medicare and Medicaid programs, and can provide any special programs or therapy the elderly person needs.

Checking reports of surveys. Reports from the State survey agency can give important clues to the health and safety conditions in the home: the Skilled Nursing Facility Survey Report, the Intermediate Care Facility Survey Report, and the Fire Safety Survey Report.

Each nursing home that participates in Medicare (as a skilled nursing facility) or in Medicaid (as a skilled nursing facility or an intermediate care facility) must be surveyed by the State at least once every 12 months to determine if it meets Federal standards. A review of these reports will show any deficiencies the facility may have.

Each report and accompanying statement of deficiencies and written comments are available to the public within 90 days following completion of the survey.

- *Medicare* survey reports are available at any local Social Security Office.
- The statements of deficiencies and written comments are available at the Social Security District Office, and public assistance agency servicing the area in which the nursing home surveyed is located.
- The State Welfare Department is responsible for establishing procedures for the disclosure of survey information for facilities participating only in the *Medicaid* program. Contact your local public assistance agency for information on the location of survey reports for skilled nursing facilities participating in Medicaid only and for reports on intermediate care facilities.

NURSING HOMES

Keep in mind, however, that no nursing home can participate in Medicare and/or Medicaid if it has serious deficiencies which place the health and safety of the patients in jeopardy. In addition, deficiencies noted on the report form must be corrected by the facility within a reasonable length of time.

Reviewing the statement of patients' rights. Ask for a copy of this statement; the home is required to make it available to the public. Note whether it covers the points required by Federal regulations as described in Part Two. During your visit, look for signs that patients' rights are actually being honored. You should also ask to see a copy of any Admission Agreement or Contract that the home may use.

CHECKING WITH THE STATE NURSING HOME OMBUDSMAN. Each State is now required by law to have a State Nursing Home Ombudsman. An important role of the ombudsman is to investigate and resolve complaints made by or on behalf of residents in nursing homes. The ombudsman is particularly concerned with any problems that may adversely affect the health, safety, welfare, and rights of nursing home residents. You may wish to check with the ombudsman to find out whether there are any serious complaints from residents in the nursing home you are considering. A listing of the State Nursing Home Ombudsman offices is in the Appendix of this publication.

TOURING THE HOME. You should be given a tour of the home by the administrator (if possible) or some other member of the staff. Look around carefully as you go, and feel free to ask questions about anything you do not understand.

General Observations. Try to see all the important areas of the home. Here are some things to look for in all areas of the nursing home:

Note the general appearance and atmosphere of the home. It should be pleasant, comfortable, attractively furnished and decorated. There should be touches that make it seem more like a home. Though the home may have a "lived-in" look, it should definitely be clean.

The home should also be reasonably free of unpleasant odors. This is a matter that requires some judgment. Where patients lack control of the bowels and bladder, *some* odors are to be expected, particularly in the early morning.

Prevention of accidents must be a major concern in nursing homes. Objects should not be left where patients may bump into

NURSING HOMES

them or trip over them. There should not be conditions that could lead to slips, such as wet spots or loose rugs on floors. In addition, nursing homes should always have devices to help patients steady themselves, such as handrails in hallways and grab bars in bathrooms and toilets.

Residents' rooms. For most residents, no part of the home is more important than their own rooms.

Visit some of the residents' rooms; they should be clean, comfortable, and pleasant. Ask about the procedures the nursing home takes to ensure that roommates are compatible.

Try to get an idea of how many beds in the home are occupied. In most areas, the good nursing homes are almost always occupied to near-capacity.

Each bedroom should have no more than four beds, a window, and access to the corridor. Mirrors in the room should be arranged for convenient use by residents in wheelchairs as well as by patients in a standing position. In rooms with more than one person, there should be fire resistant screens or curtains to ensure privacy.

In addition, each resident should have:
- an adjustable bed with a comfortable mattress and pillow
- adequate closet space (wardrobe, locker, or closet) with a clothes rod and adjustable shelf provided
- a bedside cabinet or table
- a comfortable non-folding chair
- a reading lamp
- a readily available individual bedpan, urinal, and/or washbasin and access to a lavatory or toilet room.

Each home should have enough over-bed or over-chair side tables to meet the needs of the residents. At each bed and in each toilet, bathing, and shower room, there should be within easy reach an automatic call button connected to the nearest nurses' station.

Ask how the home selects roommates. Putting two people together without considering their special interests, cultural background, and personalities can lead to conflict.

MEDICAL AND NURSING SERVICES. Because medical and nursing care are crucial to resident's welfare, you will want to find out as much about them as you can.

NURSING HOMES

If the elderly person will depend on the nursing home's physician, make a point of meeting him either at the home or later, in his office. Find out how often he visits and whether he actually sees residents, and how often he reviews their records. Ask what arrangements have been made for handling emergencies in the home and for making emergency transfers to a hospital. (You also might check with the hospital to find out their emergency procedures.)

Visit the nurses' station (the headquarters for the nursing staff). Ask for an explanation of the nurses' calling system by which residents can signal for help.

Ask to be shown the room where drugs are stored and prepared. Find out how drugs are safeguarded and who is authorized to administer them.

RESTRAINTS. On occasion, there may be a need for physical and/or chemical restraints. Restraints must be prescribed by the doctor, and should be used only when required to protect the health and safety of the patient. When a chemical restraint (medication) is used, a nurse must check the patient periodically to make sure there are no adverse side-effects. When a physical restraint is used, the patient should be monitored even more often to see that all is well, and to take care of any physical needs such as toileting. Ask about the nursing home's procedures with regard to checking on patients when restraints are used, and try to observe how the other patients seem to be faring.

Rehabilitation and activities programs. The efforts made to help residents regain their physical capacities and to provide them with satisfying recreational activities also deserve special attention.

Ask to see the schedule of events for the week. Note how often therapy sessions are scheduled and whether a variety of recreational activities is offered.

Try to see physical therapy, occupational therapy, and speech therapy in action. If this is not possible, at least visit the areas where these programs are conducted. If the therapists are on hand, make a point of talking with them. Ask to look at craft projects that residents in occupational therapy have completed or that are in progress. Watch a recreational activity in progress.

Food services. Obviously, the health and morale of residents is very much affected by the quality of the food they get. This is another area where you can rely heavily on your own experience.

NURSING HOMES

Inspect the kitchen. Although it is geared to serve a large number of people, it should be just as clean and orderly as your own kitchen at home.

Watch the kitchen staff in action for a while. They should function as a well-organized team. Look for signs that foods needing refrigeration, such as milk, cream sauces and mayonnaise, are not left standing on counter tops.

Ask to see the menus for the week. Are the meals interesting and varied? Is a snack offered at bedtime? Are between-meal snacks available during the day? Are the meal times at usually accepted hours of the day?

Ask about how special diets are handled. You should see special menus for therapeutic diets—low salt, low fat, and so on—and there should be some system for identifying patients who require these special meals.

Notice the food being prepared or served. It should be appetizing and attractive. Check whether it corresponds to the posted menu and adequate substitute food provided.

Ask to sample the food. (In some nursing homes, you may be invited to eat a meal in the dining room.) Is the food tasty? Would you be happy eating food of that quality day after day?

Watch patients eating a meal and note whether the patients appear to be enjoying the food. Are people who need it given help with eating, both in the dining room and in their own rooms? Are those who do not care for the food given something else they like better that has the same nutritional value?

MAKING FOLLOW-UP OBSERVATIONS. Consider going back for a second visit, particularly if you are unsure about anything. If you come during visiting hours, the administrator should not object. The best time to plan a second visit is during the evening hours, when there are usually fewer staff members on duty.

Take a leisurely walk through the facility, and try to determine answers to the following questions:

- Do the residents seem to receive attention in the evening?
- Are staff attitudes the same in the evening as during the day?
- Are there any evening activities for the residents?
- Does the evening staffing seem to be adequate to meet resident needs?

NURSING HOMES

Take time to chat with residents about how they feel about care in the nursing home. Their attitudes may be very revealing.

CHECKING COSTS AND OTHER ARRANGEMENTS. If all or part of the resident's bill will not be covered by the Federal insurance plans or other benefits, you will naturally be concerned about costs. Even Medicare and Medicaid do not cover all of the costs of care for residents in a nursing home.

Costs may vary from one nursing home to another. If you look carefully, you should be able to find a home that provides quality care at a reasonable price.

Charges. Unfortunately, billings are sometimes complicated, and different homes handle them in different ways. This may make it difficult to estimate what a typical month's bill will be and to compare the cost of one home with another.

Nearly all nursing homes have a basic monthly charge. Most also make other charges as well. The difficulty comes because there is no uniformity in determining which things are covered under the basic charge and which are "extras."

Usually the basic charge covers *at least* room and meals, housekeeping, linen, general nursing care, medical records services, recreation and personal care and similar services and materials that are provided equally to all patients. Generally, extra charges are made for items that vary from patient to patient.

These are extras in most nursing homes:
- Physician services, including the work of specialists like dentists, ophthalmologists, podiatrists, etc.
- Drugs and medications
- Physical therapy
- Diagnostic services such as laboratory work, x-rays, electrocardiograms, etc.
- Personal services such as telephone calls, personal laundry, beauticians and barbers.

Additional items are considered by many homes as part of the basic charge, whereas in other homes they are considered as extras. Included in this category are such items as the administration of drugs, examinations, special diets, and help with daily activities such as eating and bathing.

NURSING HOMES

Medicare will pay for items and services furnished by a SNF that are necessary for the care of the patient. Medicaid will also pay for the care and services needed by the patient. However, some items such as drugs may not be fully covered by Medicaid in some States. Under Medicare, after 20 days, there is a co-insurance amount that must be paid by the patient.

Private pay residents may be billed once for the length of a patient's stay, as a flat charge each month, or each time a service or material is provided. For example, a nursing home may make a one-time-only charge for a special mattress, may rent a wheelchair by the month, and may make a charge each time a person is given an injection or fed by hand.

Some other important matters. Here are some other financial and legal questions that should be answered.

> Will a refund be made for unused days paid in advance? It is common practice to pay the monthly charge in advance, but a person may not stay in the home for the full month. Some homes keep the full payment anyway, others make a refund for the unused days.
>
> If a resident's cash or other assets are entrusted to the home, determine how these are handled and accounted for. The resident should be given a signed receipt for all deposits, all withdrawals should be noted on a monthly or quarterly statement of funds, prepared and signed by the nursing home administrator. In this way, the patient can keep track of his or her account.
>
> Before a final choice is made, be sure you have a clear understanding about the following matters:
>
> - The daily rate, and exactly what is and what is not included in this rate.
> - The exact charges for supplies and services not included in this daily rate.
> - What will happen when personal funds are depleted and Medicaid (Title XIX) assistance is required.
> - What will happen if there is a change in the level of care needed by the patient.
> - The arrangements the facility has for pharmacy service.

NURSING HOMES

MAKING THE DECISION. Once you have visited several nursing homes and have figured out about how much they will cost, you are ready to see how they stack up against one another. In making comparisons, you will find it helpful to fill out the checklist in this booklet for each of the homes. You may find that none of the homes you are considering meets all the points described in this booklet. But keep in mind that some of the questions are more important than others, so simply adding up the "yes" and "no" answers will not give you a fool-proof basis for comparison. You must also use your own judgment. And if you are not sure how important an item is to the particular person who needs the home, a telephone call to his or her physician should help you decide.

If at all possible, do not let costs be the only factor you consider in choosing a home. The *quality* of care is critical. And by all means, let the elderly person play a part in making the decision.

MAKING THE SELECTION. For most people, finding ways to finance nursing home care is a major concern. If the elderly person does not qualify for care under Medicare or Medicaid programs, check whether his or her private health insurance covers nursing home costs. Retirement and pension plans may also include such coverage.

The contract. The nursing home may refer to this by one of several names: financial agreement, admission agreement, entrance contract, or some other term. What it amounts to is a contract between the nursing home and the patient spelling out the conditions under which the patient is accepted. The resident, or the person sponsoring him or her, will have to sign the contract before the patient is admitted and will be legally bound by what it says.

The contract should state the costs, the services included, legal responsibilities, and any other matters of a legally binding nature. Ideally, it should also include safeguards for the patient—patients' rights, grievance procedures, minimum nursing care, emergency procedures, and standards of food service.

Before you sign the contract, be sure you understand it completely. Ask the nursing home adminstrator to explain anything that is not clear. If possible, have a lawyer review the contract before you sign it.

NURSING HOMES

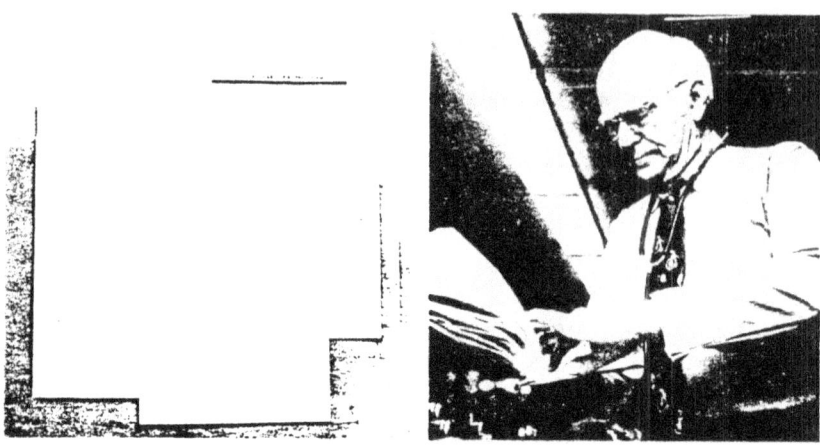

Preparing for the patient's admission. The administrator and director of social services will make arrangements with you for admitting the elderly person to the home. If the person is to be transferred from a hospital, the physician and the hospital's social worker will also be involved in the planning.

Naturally, you should do everything you can to help prepare the elderly person for entering the home. The social services director can advise you on this and may take an active part by visiting the person in advance.

To ease the transition, try to be with the elderly person on admission day and stay a few hours to help him or her get settled in.

FOLLOW UP. Once the elderly person has entered the nursing home, your responsibilities continue. Try to visit the home as often as you can. Seeing friends and relatives can be a tremendous boost to the resident's morale.

WHAT TO DO WHEN YOU HAVE A COMPLAINT. No matter how good any nursing home may be, the time may arise when you question the care, services or environment of the home. Usually, the first step in resolving such a problem is to speak directly to the nursing home administrator or to the director of nursing or of social services. If the matter is not satisfactorily settled using this approach, your next step would be to bring the problem to the attention of the Nursing Home Ombudsman in your State. Write or telephone the Nursing Home Ombudsman to discuss the grievance. The address and telephone number of the State ombudsmen are listed in the Appendix.

NURSING HOMES

PART FOUR

Checklist

The following is a checklist of important points to consider in selecting a nursing home. You should find the checklist helpful in several ways: for brushing up on things to look for and ask about before you visit a home, for referring to as you talk with staff members and tour a home, and for sizing up a home after a visit and comparing it with other homes you have visited.

There are many items on the list, because nursing homes are complex operations. To cover all the items, you may have to make additional visits or follow-up telephone calls.

Some of the items will be difficult to find out on your own, so you will probably have to ask personnel of the home.

This checklist is offered to serve as a reference guide:

The name of nursing **Home A** is _____
The name of nursing **Home B** is _____
The name of nursing **Home C** is _____

	HOME A Yes/No	HOME B Yes/No	HOME C Yes/No
Is the home certified to participate in the Medicare and Medicaid programs?	☐ ☐	☐ ☐	☐ ☐
Does the nursing home have the required current license from the State or letter of approval from a licensing agency?	☐ ☐	☐ ☐	☐ ☐
Does the administrator have a current license?	☐ ☐	☐ ☐	☐ ☐
If the person you are placing requires special services, such as rehabilitation therapy or a therapeutic diet, does the home provide them?	☐ ☐	☐ ☐	☐ ☐

NURSING HOMES

	HOME A	HOME B	HOME C
	Yes/No	Yes/No	Yes/No
Is the general atmosphere of the nursing home warm, pleasant, and cheerful?	☐ ☐	☐ ☐	☐ ☐
Is the administrator courteous and helpful?	☐ ☐	☐ ☐	☐ ☐
Are staff members cheerful, courteous, and enthusiastic?	☐ ☐	☐ ☐	☐ ☐
Do staff members show patients genuine interest and affection?	☐ ☐	☐ ☐	☐ ☐
Do residents look well cared for and generally content?	☐ ☐	☐ ☐	☐ ☐
Are residents allowed to wear their own clothes, decorate their rooms, and keep a few prized possessions on hand?	☐ ☐	☐ ☐	☐ ☐
Is there a place for private visits with family and friends?	☐ ☐	☐ ☐	☐ ☐
Is there a written statement of patient's rights? As far as you can tell, are these points being carried out?	☐ ☐	☐ ☐	☐ ☐
Do residents, other visitors, and volunteers speak favorably about the home?	☐ ☐	☐ ☐	☐ ☐

LOCATION

	HOME A	HOME B	HOME C
Is the home near family and friends?	☐ ☐	☐ ☐	☐ ☐

GENERAL PHYSICAL CONSIDERATIONS

	HOME A	HOME B	HOME C
	Yes/No	Yes/No	Yes/No
Is the nursing home clean and orderly?	☐ ☐	☐ ☐	☐ ☐

NURSING HOMES

	HOME A	HOME B	HOME C
	Yes/No	Yes/No	Yes/No
Is the home reasonably free of unpleasant odors?	☐ ☐	☐ ☐	☐ ☐
Are toilet and bathing facilities easy for handicapped patients to use?	☐ ☐	☐ ☐	☐ ☐
Is the home well-lighted?	☐ ☐	☐ ☐	☐ ☐
Are rooms well-ventilated and kept at a comfortable temperature?	☐ ☐	☐ ☐	☐ ☐

SAFETY

	HOME A	HOME B	HOME C
	Yes/No	Yes/No	Yes/No
Are wheelchair ramps provided where necessary?	☐ ☐	☐ ☐	☐ ☐
Is the nursing home free of obvious hazards, such as obstacles to patients, hazards underfoot, unsteady chairs?	☐ ☐	☐ ☐	☐ ☐
Are there grab bars in toilet and bathing facilities and handrails on both sides of hallways?	☐ ☐	☐ ☐	☐ ☐
Do bathtubs and showers have non-slip surfaces?	☐ ☐	☐ ☐	☐ ☐
Are there smoke detectors, an automatic sprinkler system, and automatic emergency lighting?	☐ ☐	☐ ☐	☐ ☐
Are there portable fire extinguishers?	☐ ☐	☐ ☐	☐ ☐
Are exits clearly marked and exit signs illuminated?	☐ ☐	☐ ☐	☐ ☐
Are exit doors unobstructed and unlocked from inside?	☐ ☐	☐ ☐	☐ ☐

NURSING HOMES

	HOME A Yes/No	HOME B Yes/No	HOME C Yes/No
Are certain areas posted with no-smoking signs? Do staff, residents, and visitors observe them?	☐ ☐	☐ ☐	☐ ☐
Is an emergency evacuation plan posted in prominent locations?	☐ ☐	☐ ☐	☐ ☐

MEDICAL, DENTAL, AND OTHER SERVICES	HOME A Yes/No	HOME B Yes/No	HOME C Yes/No
Does the home have an arrangement with an outside dental service to provide patients with dental care when necessary?	☐ ☐	☐ ☐	☐ ☐
In case of medical emergencies, is a physician available at all times, either on staff or on call?	☐ ☐	☐ ☐	☐ ☐
Does the home have arrangements with a nearby hospital for quick transfer of nursing home patients in an emergency?	☐ ☐	☐ ☐	☐ ☐
Is emergency transportation readily available?	☐ ☐	☐ ☐	☐ ☐

PHARMACEUTICAL SERVICES	HOME A Yes/No	HOME B Yes/No	HOME C Yes/No
Are pharmaceutical services supervised by a qualified pharmacist?	☐ ☐	☐ ☐	☐ ☐
Is a room set aside for storing and preparing drugs?	☐ ☐	☐ ☐	☐ ☐
Does a qualified pharmacist maintain and monitor a record of each patient's drug therapy?	☐ ☐	☐ ☐	☐ ☐

NURSING HOMES

NURSING SERVICES	HOME A	HOME B	HOME C
	Yes/No	Yes/No	Yes/No
Is at least one registered nurse (RN) or licensed pratical nurse (LPN) on duty day and night?	☐ ☐	☐ ☐	☐ ☐
Is an RN on duty during the day, seven days a week? (For skilled nursing homes)	☐ ☐	☐ ☐	☐ ☐
Does an RN serve as director of nursing services? (For skilled nursing homes)	☐ ☐	☐ ☐	☐ ☐
Are nurse or emergency call buttons located at each patient's bed and in toilet and bathing facilities?	☐ ☐	☐ ☐	☐ ☐

FOOD SERVICES	HOME A	HOME B	HOME C
	Yes/No	Yes/No	Yes/No
Is the kitchen clean and reasonably tidy? Is food needing refrigeration not left standing out on counters? Is waste properly disposed of?	☐ ☐	☐ ☐	☐ ☐
Ask to see the meal schedule. Are at least three meals served each day? Are meals served at normal hours, with plenty of time for leisurely eating?	☐ ☐	☐ ☐	☐ ☐
Are nutritious between-meal and bedtime snacks available?	☐ ☐	☐ ☐	☐ ☐
Are patients given enough food? Does the food look appetizing?	☐ ☐	☐ ☐	☐ ☐
Sample a meal. Is the food tasty and served at the proper temperature?	☐ ☐	☐ ☐	☐ ☐
Does the meal being served match the posted menu?	☐ ☐	☐ ☐	☐ ☐

NURSING HOMES

	HOME A Yes/No	HOME B Yes/No	HOME C Yes/No
Are special meals prepared for patients on therapeutic diets?	☐ ☐	☐ ☐	☐ ☐
Is the dining room attractive and comfortable?	☐ ☐	☐ ☐	☐ ☐
Do patients who need it get help in eating, whether in the dining room or in their own rooms?	☐ ☐	☐ ☐	☐ ☐

REHABILITATION THERAPY	HOME A Yes/No	HOME B Yes/No	HOME C Yes/No
Is a full-time program of physical therapy available for patients who need it?	☐ ☐	☐ ☐	☐ ☐
Are occupational therapy and speech therapy available for patients who need them?	☐ ☐	☐ ☐	☐ ☐

SOCIAL SERVICES & PATIENT ACTIVITIES	HOME A Yes/No	HOME B Yes/No	HOME C Yes/No
Are there social services available to aid patients and their families?	☐ ☐	☐ ☐	☐ ☐
Does the nursing home have a varied program of recreational, cultural, and intellectual activities for patients?	☐ ☐	☐ ☐	☐ ☐
Is there an activities coordinator on the staff?	☐ ☐	☐ ☐	☐ ☐
Is suitable space available for patient activities? Are tools and supplies provided?	☐ ☐	☐ ☐	☐ ☐
Are activities offered for patients who are relatively inactive or confined to their rooms?	☐ ☐	☐ ☐	☐ ☐

NURSING HOMES

	HOME A Yes/No	HOME B Yes/No	HOME C Yes/No
Look at the activities schedule. Are activities provided each day? Are some activities scheduled in the evenings?	☐ ☐	☐ ☐	☐ ☐
Do patients have an opportunity to attend religious services and talk with clergymen both in and outside the home?	☐ ☐	☐ ☐	☐ ☐

PATIENTS' ROOMS

	HOME A Yes/No	HOME B Yes/No	HOME C Yes/No
Does each room open onto a hallway?	☐ ☐	☐ ☐	☐ ☐
Does each room have a window to the outside?	☐ ☐	☐ ☐	☐ ☐
Does each patient have a reading light, a comfortable chair, and a closet and drawers for personal belongings?	☐ ☐	☐ ☐	☐ ☐
Is there fresh drinking water within reach?	☐ ☐	☐ ☐	☐ ☐
Is there a curtain or screen available to provide privacy for each bed whenever necessary?	☐ ☐	☐ ☐	☐ ☐
Do bathing and toilet facilities have adequate privacy?	☐ ☐	☐ ☐	☐ ☐

OTHER AREAS OF THE NURSING HOME

	HOME A Yes/No	HOME B Yes/No	HOME C Yes/No
Is there a lounge where patients can chat, read, play games, watch television, or just relax away from their rooms?	☐ ☐	☐ ☐	☐ ☐
Is a public telephone available for patients' use?	☐ ☐	☐ ☐	☐ ☐

NURSING HOMES

	HOME A Yes/No	HOME B Yes/No	HOME C Yes/No
Does the nursing home have an outdoor area where patients can get fresh air and sunshine?	☐ ☐	☐ ☐	☐ ☐

FINANCIAL AND RELATED MATTERS	HOME A Yes/No	HOME B Yes/No	HOME C Yes/No
Do the estimated monthly costs (including extra charges) compare favorably with the cost of other homes?	☐ ☐	☐ ☐	☐ ☐
Is a refund made for unused days paid for in advance?	☐ ☐	☐ ☐	☐ ☐
Are visiting hours convenient for patients and visitors?	☐ ☐	☐ ☐	☐ ☐
Are these and other important matters specified in the contract? (See page 29)	☐ ☐	☐ ☐	☐ ☐

BASIC FUNDAMENTALS OF GERIATRIC NURSING
CONTENTS

	Page
SECTION I. INTRODUCTION	1
1. General	1
2. Qualities Needed by the Specialist in Geriatric Nursing	1
3. Physiological Changes in the Geriatric Patient	2
4. Reaction of Nursing Personnel to Geriatric Patient	3
5. Additional Time Required by the Patient	3
II. GENERAL NURSING CARE MEASURES	4
6. Bathing and Skin Care	4
7. Sleep and Rest	4
8. Clothing	5
9. Exercise and Recreation	5
10. Elimination	5
11. Enemas	6
12. Nutrition	6
13. Communication	6
14. Diseases of Old Age	6
15. Needs of Geriatric Patient	7
16. Special Precautions	9
17. Role of the Health Nurse in Geriatric Care	9

BASIC FUNDAMENTALS OF GERIATRIC NURSING

Section I. INTRODUCTION

1. General

a. *Definition of the Aged Person.* Chronological age does not make anyone young or old. Some people are young in spirit at age 90; others are old at 21. However, the chronological age of 65 is arbitrarily considered the dividing point between the middle-aged and the aged or old person. This is the age when retirement from active employment generally takes place and when Old Age and Survivors Insurance (Social Security) benefits commence.

b. *Geriatric Nursing.* Geriatric nursing can be defined as caring for persons aged 65 or older. It cuts across many other fields of nursing, incorporating basic principles of nursing care. The specialist caring for a geriatric patient will utilize principles found in medical-surgical nursing, gynecological nursing, and psychiatric nursing, to mention only a few. Geriatric nursing in many ways is like any other type of nursing, yet in other ways it is different or special. What makes geriatric nursing special or different and how the specialist should act and react when caring for the elderly patient is the purpose of this chapter. Largely, the change lies in the approach, attitude, and personal warmth of nursing personnel, plus a knowledge of the aging process.

c. *Importance of Geriatric Nursing.* The ability to provide adequate and safe nursing services to the older age group is becoming of paramount importance. Between **2000,** and **2030** the percentage of the U.S. population over 65 years of age is expected to quintuple. More and more, elderly persons are found both within the civilian and the military hospital environment; this is expected to continue and even expand. It is a well-known fact that people are living longer. Medical science has made giant strides in the maintenance of health and the prevention of disease, as well as in curing disease and rehabilitating persons following disease or injury.

2. Qualities Needed by the Specialist in Geriatric Nursing

a. A specialist who assists with a geriatric patient will need to be emotionally stable and slow to anger, a condition known as maturity. The aged may be talkative, secretive, hostile, rude, and childish, but the specialist must not take their remarks personally. He must try to understand their behavior and react in a nonjudgmental manner.

b. The specialist must express sincere interest and affection for the geriatric patient. Old people recognize and detest insincerity. All nursing personnel should be kind, tolerant, and patient, but geriatric nursing personnel *must* be. These qualities come only when you have gained true respect for yourself; respect will then be given to others.

c. The specialist must also have empathy (a projection of one's own personality into the problems and personality of another; a feeling *with* someone). If a specialist can imagine that he has lost his job, lost his friends, lost his sensory perceptions, lost his home, lost his ability to speak fluently, lost his health, and lost his self-esteem, then he can begin to understand the disagreeable stubborn outbursts of an old person. He must recognize that hostility may be an expression of fear, and stubbornness may be an expression of insecurity. He must also recognize the embarrassment that would follow the failure to do even a simple task for oneself.

d. The specialist cannot become emotionally involved with the patient. Life can be prolonged, but death always awaits the geriatric patient. It requires a special quality to show affection for these old people and yet maintain a realistic acceptance that death will surely come.

Table 1. Physiological Changes

System	Changes	Results in
Skeletal	Degenerative changes in joints. Decalcifieation-"mineral starvation" or demineralization	Pain and stiffness in joint. Fractures.
Muscular	Less muscular activity.	Slumped posture; sagging abdominal muscles; contractures.
Skin-Integumentary	Becomes dry; wrinkled, less elastic. Less oils produced. Baldness. Increased pigmentation.	Traumatized easily. Susceptible to deeubitus ulcers.
Circulatory	Degeneration of elastic tissues in blood vessels; thinning of middle layer of arterial wall; deposition of metabolic substances such as calcium and cholesterol on inner layer of arterial wall.	Impaired circulation; slower healing.
Respiratory	Rib cage rigid and less elastic; atrophy of respiratory muscles; lungs smaller; bronchioles less elastic; alveoli larger and less elastic with inner walls; vital capacity reduced.	Lowered efficiency of respiratory system.
Digestive	Less muscle tone; less mobility; less absorption of food; mucous membrane thinner; loss of tone in supportive structures.	Elimination problem; malnutrition; intestinal tissue traumatized.
Urinary	Efficiency of glomeruli reduced; muscular portion of ureter, bladder, and urethra less elastic; loss of tone of supportive structure; less blood supply.	Tissues easier traumatized and subject to infection. Reduced efficiency of urinary system.

e. The specialist must make observations for the nurse and doctor, as he will be with the patient more than they will.

3. Physiological Changes in the Geriatric Patient

The process of aging begins at birth and stops only with death. It is a very gradual process, yet the changes occur in a fairly predictable pattern, with the rate of change varying from one individual to another. It is a period that is often marked by mental confusion and vagueness. The specialist must consider this confusion and help the patient as much as possible. He must also be aware that the old person's body has undergone many other changes. The physiological changes that are seen in the geriatric patient can be generally classified as loss of elasticity in tissues and a general slowing down of the physiologic process. Table 1 illustrates some of the major changes.

4. Reaction of Nursing Personnel to Geriatric Patient

a. Some nursing service personnel may express displeasure when assigned to give care to aged people, often making such comments as "I'd much rather take care of an active duty soldier than that old retired sergeant," or "I just don't know how to handle old people." But retired sergeants or old people in general are not a group unto themselves; they are merely people who have grown old as everyone must do. As with any other person, however, they have certain basic needs, and these needs must be met if the optimum benefit from hospitalization is to be realized. Everyone needs recognition, security, and love. The nursing care plan should recognize these needs and try to satisfy them as nursing care is given.

Table . 2 Rules for Care of the Aged

DO-	DO NOT-
Treat as an individual.	Do not call old people "grandma" or "grandpa."
Call by name such as Sergeant Brown or Mrs. Green.	Do not stick to the procedure just for the procedure sake.
Be tolerant, patient, and kind.	Do not shout.
Speak slowly and distinctly.	Do not do *everything* for the patient.
Help the patient to help himself.	Do not ignore so-called minor complaints.
Be extremely observant.	Do not try to change lifelong habits of eating or sleeping.
Be optimistic.	

b. As the medical specialist cares for an aged patient, he must remember that the patient is a product of his heredity and long years of environmental pressures. The so-called, well-adjusted older person was probably a well-adjusted adult and child; whereas the so-called poorly adjusted older person who is garrulous at times and seemingly unreasonable was probably a poorly adjusted adult and child. It must be emphasized here that the habits of a lifetime will not be changed lightly or willingly; therefore, changes should be required only when absolutely necessary. *For example,* if an old person is used to having coffee at 5 o'clock every morning, he should be given the coffee at the hospital. Any adjustments that must be made should be made by the specialist, not the patient.

5. Additional Time Required by the Patient

a. The admission of an aged person on a busy ward can be disruptive. Routines geared to the adult or younger patient just do not meet the needs of the geriatrics patient. Adjustment of the routine and personnel is not without difficulty, but if the medical specialist is to fulfill his responsibility of providing nursing care, it must be done. Older patients cannot and should not be rushed, particularly in the morning. An older patient will take almost twice the time, for example, to prepare for breakfast as the younger patient. As medical specialists, you must be aware of the time involved and plan accordingly.

b. Many times it will seem easier and quicker to do something for the patient, rather than let him do it for himself, because it takes him so long. However, oversolicitous care and too much waiting on a patient will force him into a dependent role, a role he does not want and one that is incompatible with a healthy outlook on life. Avoid the temptation to take over. The aim of nursing care is to permit the patient to do as much for himself as he can, with only a minimum of assistance from nursing personnel. His small accomplishments will mean a lot to him.

Section II. GENERAL NURSING CARE MEASURES

6. Bathing and Skin Care

a. Older people do not need to bathe or be bathed daily. In fact, some medical geriatric specialists believe that once or twice weekly is sufficient. As a person ages, the skin dries because less oil is produced. Too frequent bathing might lead to skin irritation. However, areas that are soiled are bathed as needed.

b. If at all possible, the patient should be placed in a tub.

CAUTION

An elderly patient is always assisted to get in and out of a tub.

A tub bath provides an excellent opportunity to exercise all of his joints, as well as make him feel more comfortable. If getting in a tub is not possible, a wooden chair or stool should be placed in the shower or stall and the spray shower used. During the bath, whether in the tub or shower, the patient should be afforded privacy. A call light or bell should be in easy reach, and you should check on him frequently. If you cannot leave a patient because of safety reasons, do not look at him directly, but give the appearance of looking somewhere else in order to spare him embarrassment. If a patient becomes ill during a tub bath, pull the plug in the tub first and look after him. Do not leave him alone; wait for help.

c. If a patient is confined to bed, a bed bath once or twice a week, supplemented by partial bed baths and frequent massage to pressure points (but *not* to extremities) is sufficient. Since aged skin is easily traumatized, massage must be gentle. Use of alcohol should be avoided since it will tend to dry already dry skin. Use of a lanolin-rich lotion, particularly to the pressure point such as heels, elbows, and buttocks, will help. Extremities are not usually massaged because of the danger of disturbing blood clots.

d. Toenails and fingernails need careful attention. When possible, the geritric patient should be encouraged to do his own fingernails. Care of the toenails will probably have to be done by the specialist. Cutting nails or clipping cuticles too short must be avoided. If the toenails are long and horny, the physician should be informed since the services of a podiatrist may be indicated.

CAUTION

Never cut the toenails of a *diabetic* patient without a doctor's order. A break in the skin on the toe of a diabetic patient could lead to an amputation.

e. As a part of the daily routine, men should be encouraged and assisted, if necessary, to shave and to comb their hair. Use of an aromatic aftershave lotion can do much to raise the morale, especially if someone comments on it. Women, likewise, should be encouraged to fix their hair and put on makeup if they usually use it. If patients are unable to do for themselves, then the specialist should attend to these matters.

7. Sleep and Rest

a. The aged person needs warm sleeping garments and warm lightweight covers. A bed with adjustable height should be used, whenever available. If only a standard hospital bed is available, a footstool should be provided for the patient. He should be as comfortable as possible since he does not sleep as soundly as the younger patient. He will often wander up and down the ward corridors in the middle of the night. Because of this, there should be sufficient night personnel on duty and sufficient light for the patient's safety. Sonu patients will need side rails. A night snack, a glass of warm milk, or early morning coffee will help keep them more contented. Since old people sleep less at night, they tend to take naps during the day. A comfortable chair for them to doze in may rest them more than getting in and out of bed. (In fact, the exertion required for them to get into bed may wake them up.) A tap bell should always be placed near the chair when a patient is sitting up, so that he may use it if needed.

  b. More rest is needed by the geriatric patient, yet too much rest can be dangerous, if not fatal. If the doctor permits, get the patient out of bed into a chair or a wheel chair at least daily. This not only aids him physiologically, but also improves his emotional outlook by providing a change of environment.

8. Clothing

Part of any admission routine is usually to have the patient remove his own clothing and wear hospital attire. In some situations, it is necessary and desirable to wear hospital pajamas, but to the older patient, loss of his clothing may mean another step down the road of dependence. Sometimes hospital routines must be bent some to allow, *for example,* the patient to wear his "long John 's" as pajamas, if that is what he is accustomed to wearing-provided, of course, that he changes them and that either he or his family can care for them. Most older patients will dislike robes; they seem too much like sleeping garments to them. Women will like cotton smocks and men some type of shirt and loose slacks. They will often insist on long underwear-and they are right to do so. It is warmer and prevents skin surfaces from touching which, in turn, prevents chafing and soreness. At all times, clothing for old people should be soft, warm, and easily put on or cared for. Their morale will also be helped by color and style.

9. Exercise and Recreation

  a. Exercise. Motion and exercise are important aids to circulation of blood and of lymph. It also aids elimination. Inexperienced personnel may be afraid that exercise may hurt the patient; the opposite is true. The aged patient is rarely ever put on complete bedrest. A comfortable rocking chair may be sufficient exercise; however, the doctor will order the most beneficial exercise possible. The nursing care plan should include instructions about exercise or ambulation.

  b. Recreation. Old people need to be kept busy. Younger patients, if treated on the ward, can be utilized to interest the older patient in doing some activity, even if it is only talking to the geriatric patient. If possible, a dayroom or a separate room should be set aside for recreational activities. Since old people tire easily and often have limited powers of concentration, these activities must be limited to things that do not confuse or tire them. Games, religious services, and entertainment should be short. Then other factors enter

- Cost is important. Old people are generally on limited budgets.
- Projects should have a goal-not just be "busy" -perhaps a display, a sale, contest, newspaper coverage, or art show.
- Projects must be simple and individual enough so that each patient can do something. Remember some will be confused, some can work only under directions, some have trembling hands.
- Projects must be safe.

Some suggestions for recreation are group singing (use old familiar songs generally), drawing or painting pictures, dancing, knitting or sewing by hand (even men may enjoy this), quilting, checkers, dominoes, and puzzles.

10. Elimination

  a. Bowel movements are one of the primary concerns of the elderly. Evacuation *does* become a problem with advancing age. Muscle tone decreases; there is less ability to chew and therefore less bulk in the diet; and exercise is limited. Regularity is important. The specialist can check to find out when the patient usually has a bowel movement. The patient may be accustomed to sitting on a commode for long periods of time. If at all possible, try to maintain his routine and schedule. The specialist should watch closely for signs of impaction such as dribbling diarrhea and notify the nurse if this occurs. In addition, elderly patients need bulk in their diet (whole grain cereals, leafy vegetables, fruit pulps and skins; these must be cooked thoroughly or chopped if patient has chewing difficulties). Often 5 or 6 prunes in the morning are sufficient to cause a bowel movement, but individual tolerances differ greatly. Some have found their own solution; let them use it, unless contraindicated. Medication for bulk may also be ordered by the doctor. Follow directives for giving this medicine carefully.

WARNING

Be sure to answer signal lights promptly. Older people often cannot wait, especially to urinate. Older male patients may feel more secure if allowed to keep a urinal in the bed or on a chair nearby.

b. Prostate trouble is common among old men. Early symptoms which appear very gradually are frequency, difficulty in initiating the flow, and difficulty in maintaining the flow. Hematuria and the symptoms of cystitis may also occur. Many malignancies occur here, so be sure to report incipient trouble.

11. Enemas

Older people need enemas more often than younger people but, if used too often, they will interfere with normal bowel movements and wash out the mucus that lubricates the colon. Enemas are given as for other adults but a bedpan or commode should be at hand as old people cannot always control their bowel movements.

12. Nutrition

Eating should be an enjoyable experience. Pleasant conversation, a neat area, and adequate time are essentials for this enjoyment. The food that can be eaten depends on the condition of the teeth. Baby food with added seasonings is used in some cases. Proteins are essential. Also, old people are as apt as children to swallow pieces of bone or gristle and choke. They should be given small servings on an attractive tray, with perhaps a flower, a special name card, and a colorful napkin. If their food must be cut up, do so before serving them to avoid chilling the food and also to avoid embarrassment to the patient. (He may even refuse to feed himself because of his shaking hand. If this happens, try giving him only one food at a time.) Soups and liquids are easier to handle in a lightweight cup from which he can drink. He will probably need help to open such things as milk cartons and individual packets. Whether or not he feeds himself, note what he eats and how much. The specialist should offer fluid at frequent intervals to the elderly patient since the patient may not be able to help himself. Make sure if the patient has dentures that they are in his mouth at meal time. The patient may be too forgetful or too confused to ask for them.

13. Communication

a. The older patient may have to be hospitalized at a time when his speaking and hearing ability are beginning to fail. He needs to communicate badly but may not be aware of his difficulty. He may accuse you of mumbling. He may and often does misunderstand the doctor. You will have to explain to him repeatedly as he will also forget what he is told. He may learn to cover up for his failure to hear by nodding, smiling, and pretending. This is quite common. You might ask him to tell you what you said. Above all, be patient.

b. Deafness can be suspected when there is a loss of interest in group activity, in what you say, and in other people; when he attempts to lip read or seems to hear better when he can see your face; and when he apparently ignores orders or suggestions.

c. Remember that communication may be difficult with the aged person even when he can hear-probably 50 years lie between you. You even have different standards; in your world of casual exposure, you may not realize that exposed knees can embarrass an old woman. You think of hospitals as a place where you go to get well; to the old, hospitals are places where you go to die. Be sure that you are really communicating what you want him to know or do.

14. Diseases of Old Age

Some of the diseases of old age are shown in table 3.

15. Needs of Geriatric Patient

The geriatric patient needs all of the following:
- Friends and family
- Maximum self-determination
- Privacy
- Individual expression
- Personal dignity
- New experiences
- Comfort and safety

Most of all, he needs to feel needed.

Table 3. Some Diseases and Conditions of Old Age

Disease or condition	What it does and what specialist may notice	Suggestions to specialist
Arteriosclerosis (hardening of the arteries).	Interferes with sight, speech, and circulation of the aged. Causes forgetfulness, particularly of recent events; changes in personality.	Be sure to repeat instructions many times in a slow, calm, deliberate manner. Patient who "runs away" may have just gone for a walk and forgot where to go. Be patient, and do not scold.
Eyes-Cataracts	Results in dimming of vision, progressing into blindness. Has difficulty in reading small print.	Have a stronger light for reading. Give large print for reading matter. Report any complaint referable to eyes to the nurse such as spots before eyes, burning sensation, tearing. If patient has surgery, be alert for unusual reaction to sedative. If eyes are bandaged, always announce your presence.
Ears-deafness	Makes communication difficult and may cause the patient to withdraw.	Speak slowly and deliberately.
Osteoarthritis	Causes pain on motion and swelling of the joints. Patient is afraid to move.	TCL is essential but do not encourage self-pity. Change position frequently, if bedfast. Encourage movement of all joints.
Fractures	Causes immobility of patient. May mean loss of independence, invalidism, or death to the patient.	Encourage patient to do as much for self as possible. Ambulate as soon as doctor permits. Change position frequently. If casted, watch for development of pressure points. Report to nurse or doctor any swelling, cyanosis, or blanching of skin.
Skin-Loss of sensation	Causes patient to tolerate pressure that would cause younger persons to turn to relieve pressure. Skin may turn red.	Report any redness of skin to doctor or nurse. See that the patient turns frequently. Massage only on doctor's orders. It is dangerous to massage extremities, particularly if patient complains of pain, because it might result in an embolus.

Condition	Description	Care
Pruritis	Results from loss of oil. Causes intense itching. Results in excoriation of skin.	Use lanolin-rich lotion; bathe less frequently.
Arteriosclerotic heart disease.	Causes multiple small clots, which interfere with circulation to the heart muscle. Symptoms of cardiac failure, such as shortness of breath, fatigue, dependent edema.	Use slow motions. Allow patient to rest the moment he feels tired. Patient may breathe or sleep better when head is elevated.
Peripheral vascular disease	Decreases circulation to extremities because the circulatory system breaks down. Patient may complain of cold feet, numbness, tingling, or loss of feeling.	Use loose fitting socks or booties in bed. Use patient's shoes or slippers with firm soles if out of bed. Keep feet clean; soak as a part of bath.
Cerebrovascular Accidents (CVA).	Results in strange behavior, dizzy spells, forgetfulness, and confusion. Aphasia (loss of speech) and paralysis may occur.	Encourage patient to do as much as possible for self. If aphasic, talk to patient, not about him; he may understand more than he shows. Have patient use pencil and paper as a means of communication if possible. Protect against injury; *for example,* support in wheel chair and use bed side rails.
Cancer	Can result in mutilating surgery. May be cured. Often seen as a terminal case. Because of this, the word can cause extreme fear and anxiety. Patient may be apathetic or extremely anxious.	Attend to patient's physical needs as promptly as possible. Keep as comfortable as possible through nursing measures: turn frequently, give back rubs, and give medication for pain when requested by patient. Listen to patient; you may be his "sounding board." Encourage family to visit frequently.
Diabetics	Causes poor circulation and slow healing of injuries. A small injury to foot may result in amputation.	Encourage him to eat all food on tray, report what is left to nurse. Old people may act like children when confronted with a diet. They may get candy bars or refuse to eat. Foot care is extremely important. Keep extremely clean; give immediate care to any broken area; cut nails and fingernails only on doctor's orders and then very carefully. Check shoes for proper fit; hose or socks must not have mends or ridges.

Disease or condition	What it does and what specialist may notice	Suggestions to specialist
Pneumonia	Often causes light cough, drowsiness, and apathy. Patient may not appear as ill as he is.	Keep patient comfortable, often in a low Fowler's position. Put a pillow against the lower back or elevate the head of the bed on shock blocks. May be more comfortable in a chair but avoid exerting him, as pneumonia places a strain on the heart.
Tuberculosis	Causes cough and sputum. Common among elderly people, especially men. May not look as sick as he really is.	Teach him how to protect others but make allowance for his habits. If he will not use tissues, get soft rags that can be burned. While patient is in the hospital, he should be referred to the Health Nurse for contact investigation and for patient and/or family education on tuberculosis. If he is returned home, the Health Nurse should continue involvement in the case, checking him and his family by periodic contact followup and public health supervision of patient and family in the home.

16. Special Precautions
- Be especially alert to any confusion following sedation. Old people often have adverse reactions to sedatives and to medications given for pain.
- If a heating pad or hot water bottle is ordered by the physician, check frequently for condition of skin. Older people have a tendency to poor circulation and decreased sensation in their extremities. The patient may not realize the heating pad is too hot until he is burned.
- If postural drainage is necessary, try merely elevating the foot of the bed first as this may be enough, or put the patient's head at the foot of bed, placing the side with the affected lung uppermost and raising the knee gatch. He must be watched closely as he may not be able to tolerate it. Unless specifically ordered, the elderly patient is never placed crosswise on the bed with his head resting on the floor.
- If oxygen is ordered, give the geriatric patient special assurance. He may think this is a last resort and that he is dying.
- Insure that aged patients get frequent periods of exercise alternating with frequent periods of rest.
- Insure that he has proper ventilation. This is essential, since the decreased chest expansion and impaired circulation decrease the oxygen supply to the tissues. Do not put a geriatric patient in a draft, however.

17. Role of the Health Nurse in Geriatric Care

Because the older patient's illness may be a long one, with alternating periods of hospitalization and home care; because he may be alone and need special guidance; because of the need for special instructions to his family, the Health Nurse is usually consulted in health problems involving geriatrics. The time of her involvement will be decided by the doctor or nuise, but it will probably be *before the patient returns home*. The specialist should furnish her with any information requested.

www.ingramcontent.com/pod-product-compliance
Lightning Source LLC
Chambersburg PA
CBHW081823300426
44116CB00014B/2468